Working It Out

Working It Out

Using Exercise in Psychotherapy

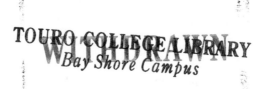

Kate F. Hays

AMERICAN PSYCHOLOGICAL ASSOCIATION

WASHINGTON, DC

Published by
American Psychological Association
750 First Street, NE
Washington, DC 20002

Copies may be ordered from
APA Order Department
P.O. Box 92984
Washington, DC 20090-2984

In the U.K., Europe, Africa, and the Middle East, copies may be ordered from
American Psychological Association
3 Henrietta Street
Covent Garden, London
WC2E 8LU England

Typeset in Meridien by Harlowe Typography, Cottage City, MD

Printer: Bookcrafters, Chelsea, MI
Jacket Designer: Minker Design, Bethesda, MD
Technical/Production Editor: Eleanor Inskip

Library of Congress Cataloging-in-Publication Data

Hays, Kate F.
    Working it out : using exercise in psychotherapy / Kate F. Hays.
       p.   cm.
    Includes bibliographical references and indexes.
    ISBN 1-55798-592-8 (case : alk. paper)
    1. Exercise therapy. 2. Exercise—Psychological aspects.
  3. Mental health promotion. I. Title.
  RC489.E9H39 1999
  616.89'1—DC21   99-18204
                                        CIP

British Library Cataloguing-in-Publication Data
A CIP record is available from the British Library.

Printed in the United States of America
First Edition

To
Lora Hays,
who continues to be a role model for the
synergy of mental and physical activity.

Contents

PREFACE   *ix*

INTRODUCTION   *xi*

I

BASICS OF THE BODY–MIND CONNECTION

1   "Affective Beneficence": Exercise
     and Well Being   3

2   The Client, Exercise, and the Therapist   11

3   Theory and Practice in the Therapeutics
     of Exercise   21

II

CHOOSING EXERCISE AS A THERAPEUTIC TOOL

4   The Process of Change   37

5   The Pragmatics of Exercise Initiation
     and Maintenance   47

6   Walking the Walk While Talking the Talk:
     Exercise with Clients   59

III

THE PSYCHOLOGICAL BENEFITS OF EXERCISE
WITH SPECIFIC POPULATIONS

7   Overcoming Inertia: Exercise and Depression   75

8   Calm in Motion: Exercise for Anxiety   87

9   Staying Sane: Exercise and Stress Management, Self-Esteem, and Mastery   97

10   Loss and Gain: Exercise and Eating   107

11   Pacing Oneself: Exercise and Substance Abuse Recovery   119

12   "Burning Off Negative Thoughts": Exercise for People With Chronic Mental Illness   129

13   From Being Alive to Feeling Alive: Trauma Survivor Empowerment   137

14   Healthy and Strong: Exercise and Recovery From Medical Illness   147

15   Oxymorons and Stereotypes: Exercise and Diversity Issues   153

16   Having Fun: Exercise Across the Life Span   167

17   Beyond the Game: Athletes With Emotional Problems   177

IV

CAVEATS AND BOUNDARIES

18   When Bad Things Happen to Good Sports: The Consequences of Overuse   191

19   Being Fit: Ethical Issues Relevant to Exercise and Therapy   203

20   The Next Steps: Education, Training, and Marketing   215

GLOSSARY: EXERCISE AND SPORT PSYCHOLOGY TERMS   *225*

APPENDIX A: EXERCISE AND SPORT PSYCHOLOGY DEVELOPMENT PLAN   *229*

APPENDIX B: A BRIEF HISTORY OF EXERCISE AND SPORT PSYCHOLOGY   *239*

APPENDIX C: EXERCISE HISTORY, MOTIVATION INVENTORY, AND EXERCISE PLAN   *243*

REFERENCES   *247*

AUTHOR INDEX   *267*

SUBJECT INDEX   *273*

ABOUT THE AUTHOR   *281*

Preface

"What business are you really in?" Until I read those words of John Naisbitt's some years ago in *Megatrends*, I had thought I was a psychologist. Reflecting, it became clear to me that my business was really one of translation. My task was to bridge the gaps between what is known in one realm and unknown in another. At an individual level, that may mean translating the unconscious into the conscious, clarifying core constructs, or linking past suffering to present pain to future options. Among families, groups, or communities, my task has been to translate psychological concepts in ways that can be of practical use to people. My assumption throughout has been that the more that people know and understand, the more flexibility they have in the decisions they make and the ways they choose to lead their lives.

When I came to sport psychology, I was well launched in my career as a clinical psychologist. But the pull to translate has remained with me. What fascinated me at a personal level was the greater access I had to my own internal processes when I exercised—being able to translate myself to myself. But more, it was the various external interrelations that piqued my involvement. I was endlessly fascinated by the interconnections between exercise and sport, between mind and body, between researchers and practitioners—and all of this in regard to how what I was learning might be of interest to other psychotherapists.

After writing a number of articles and book chapters, I knew, viscerally, that a book of some sort was my next step. Wisely, I waited until the right topic appeared in my head.

In the midst of writing the fourth in a four-part *Psychotherapy Bulletin* series for psychologists on the many facets of exercise and sport psychology, I had an inspired thought: A few more chapters like these and I'll have a book. "Piece o' cake." On such optimism is a book begun.

That initial vision has sustained me, nonetheless. And in the process I have been inspired and encouraged by many, many people. I now am firmly convinced that it takes a village to write a book. The village of my mind starts with my elders. Through fortuity and high-order serendipity, I developed lifelong and knowledge-engaging mentorships and friendships with colleagues, including initially, Michael Sachs, Carole Oglesby, Bonnie Berger, Bill Morgan, Dick Suinn, and the late and much-missed Steve Heyman. As I have become involved in the life and work of two sport psychology organizations (the Division of Exercise and Sport Psychology of the American Psychological Association and the Association for the Advancement of Applied Sport Psychology), that list of connections has exponentiated—and continues to fortify me. My village has grown huge. If I were to attempt to list its inhabitants, I would no doubt exclude someone whose good will and involvement has assisted me greatly, particularly in this enormous undertaking that becomes synthesized into the simple phrase, writing a book. My good friends and acquaintances have provided a reference here, an obscure article there, their curiosity and confidence. I hope and trust that they know how invaluable that has been.

Here, I will limit myself to thanking those who have most tangibly assisted in this process. First, I extend gratitude to those who, each in their own way, knew my book before I did: Linda Campbell, Pat DeLeon, and Gary VandenBos. The questionnaire participants, some of whose voices are heard throughout this book, helped me develop and elaborate the vision. Although their identities are masked here, my clients were willing to expand their physical and mental horizons. And Charlie Brown, Karen Cogan, Sandra Foster, Joan Joesting-Mahoney, Lynda Koenig, Andy Meyers, Greg Mondin, Shane Murphy, Wes Sime, Rob Smith, and Tim Wildman each took on the challenge of reading and helpfully commenting on some part or all of this book. Margaret Schlegel and Ed Meidenbauer, editorial midwives of the finest calibre, have made the birthing of this book a pleasure. And finally, I wish to express deep gratitude to Jeff Brown, whose generosity of time, spirit, red pen, and praise have nourished me.

Introduction

A sound mind in a sound body is a short but full description of a happy state in this world. He that has these two has little more to wish for; and he that wants either of them will be little the better for anything else.

John Locke
Some Thoughts Concerning Education

In our work as practitioners, we are the keepers of hope. Our task is to honor our clients' pain while appreciating their potential. Thus, it is appealing when we encounter a means for counteracting the negative spiral or vicious cycle with which many clients present themselves for therapy. Helping clients achieve an interaction of mind and body is one such synergistic delicious cycle. This relationship is spiraling, helical, or even weblike, one effect in turn becoming the cause of another.

Moving our bodies is one way to help move our minds—just as, in turn, our thoughts and feelings can alter our use of our bodies. In the broadest sense of the term, working out allows us to stretch not only our physical but also our mental muscles. The persistence of physical activity strengthens intrapsychic endurance. Rhythmic routine soothes and smooths our thoughts. The shared camaraderie of physical activity connects us with others. The unification of mind and body connects us with ourselves. Exercise allows us to resolve, that is, to work out, concerns, crises, and conflicts.

This book is intended to inspire mental health professionals to bring to their work a clearer understanding of, interest in, and enthusiasm for exercise in the process of recovery from mental or emotional problems. It blends theory, research, and practice experience. Reading, reflecting, and acting on these concepts should be an engaging rather than a static process. The primary theme directs psychotherapists toward the value of exercise in the treatment of most psychiatric conditions. A subtext supports psychotherapists' exercise, for their own well-being as well as that of their clients. A third aspect weaves in practice issues: practitioner recommendations, means of integrating concepts from exercise and sport psychology into one's practice, and a taste of the myriad alternate and elaborated possibilities that such practice can offer. In the next few pages, I describe my personal experience with exercise and the results of a survey of other therapists who exercise. I conclude this Introduction with an overview of the contents of the book.

Practicing What We Preach

Once people have experienced the best-for-them match with exercise, they come to genuinely love to exercise and get pleasure out of moving their bodies. In my late 30s, I started running. I underwent an immediate, 24-hour conversion to the pleasure of this activity. This passion was approximately 180° opposite of the assumptions I had previously made about running (i.e., boring, compulsive, time wasting, and tiring). Being an introspective and intellectualized sort of person, I soon realized that what most captivated me was my sense that I thought differently when I ran. It took me a few more years to recognize that this discovery was not mere coincidence. My life at the time was in personal crisis, and running allowed me to think through my situation in different ways. More accurately, I less thought about it than let novel and constructive solutions and resolutions emerge. It was indeed powerful and creative stress management.

From my own experience with exercise and its effects I developed an interest in exercise and sport psychology. As I began to read and understand the relevant literature, it occurred to me that some of my personal observations and conclusions might be generalizable:

- Times of crisis, when clients come into therapy, are often optimal moments to introduce change, such as exercise.

■ The correct person-to-exercise match cannot necessarily be predicted. Sometimes serendipity happens; sometimes people need to venture out to find what works for them.

■ Certain profound body–mind interactions occur that do not have any name but are nonetheless real. Physiological access to psychological understanding is one such process.

Since then, I have had conversations with numerous other people whose exercise experience has encompassed these thought or mood alterations. Along with feeling validated, I have wondered: If these people are therapists, in what ways does their own experience affect their interactions with clients about exercising?

Surveys of therapists indicate that 50%–75% report regular physical exercise as one aspect of their own self-care (Barrow, English, & Pinkerton, 1987; Burks & Keeley, 1989; Coster & Schwebel, 1997; Mahoney, 1997; Royak-Schaler & Feldman, 1984). These same surveys also have addressed the question of whether therapists recommend exercise to their clients. For the most part, recommending exercise on a consistent basis occurs with great infrequency (Barrow, English, & Pinkerton, 1987; Burks & Keeley, 1989). "It is apparent that most therapists believe in the efficacy of regular exercise and engage in various forms of physical activity, but few recommend exercise to their clients" (McEntee & Halgin, 1996, p. 50). As with other health care providers, such as physicians, certified nurse midwives, and physician assistants (Pender, Sallis, Long, & Calfas, 1994), therapists are more likely to recommend exercise if they themselves exercise (Royak-Schaler & Feldman, 1984). "Most pro-exercise responses came from therapists whose beliefs and practices were largely self-informed; people who had benefitted personally from exercise were more likely to want to relate those experiences to their clients" (McEntee & Halgin, 1996, p. 57).

Questionnaire on Exercise: The Survey and Results

Out of my own interest in the qualitative aspects of exercise among therapists, I developed an exploratory *Questionnaire on Exercise*. Designed to examine the function of exercise in the lives of mental health practitioners, it sought information in three general areas: practitioners' own exercise patterns, history, and thoughts; their recommendation of exercise to clients; and the use of exercising with clients during therapy.

With regard to therapists' own direct experience, I was curious whether those who exercised described the widely reported positive effects of exercise (e.g., well-being, good health, weight management, and socialization). Furthermore, I wanted to hear whether there were particular modes of thinking (e.g., increased creativity) that occurred when therapists exercised. In terms of recommending exercise to clients, I asked the following: Under what circumstances do psychotherapists recommend exercise to their clients? What criteria do they use? What benefits do they observe? What risks are they concerned about? And finally, since there is a dearth of such information, I wanted to find out more about therapists' use of exercise with clients during therapy—frequency, potential benefits, and possible risks.

Essentially, I was hoping to capture in written form the meat or essence of some of my prior conversations. At various professional meetings, both local and national, as well as through relevant electronic mail lists, I sought responses from interested practitioners. The responses reported here are from 66 therapists who exercise, 34 women and 32 men. Most were in their mid-20s to their mid-50s, with a median age of about 45. Professionally, the respondents were primarily psychologists, although 15 of the total were psychiatric social workers, psychiatrists, licensed pastoral psychotherapists, and counselors. The voices of a number of these survey respondents can be heard throughout this book, in relevant sidebars.

THERAPISTS' OWN EXERCISE PATTERNS

All but a few of the respondents currently exercise and have been doing so for a wide range of time, 6 months to 30 years. Additionally, a wide range of forms and types, frequency, intensity and duration of exercise was reported, illustrating these therapists' versatility and overall love of movement. Descriptively, much of the exercise is rhythmic, noncompetitive, and predictable, characteristics that Berger (1994) has described as maximizing the psychological benefits of exercise. Approximately one fifth of the men, but only a few women, mentioned competition and competitive training.

Exercise is a predictable part of these people's day, rather than a haphazard experience. Most described a typical daily or weekly pattern (e.g., calisthenics for 30 minutes alone, 5 days a week, or a daily hour of aerobic activity—cycling, running, or swimming—and 30 minutes working out with weights 3 times a week). For those who engage in competitive sport, variations occur in relation to the competitive season.

A wide range of types of exercise, frequency, intensity, and duration was reported. One therapist runs daily on step equipment, alone, for 15 minutes first thing in the morning. A psychologist reported running about 50 miles a week, mostly alone, works out once a week for about an hour and a half with a group, lifts weights daily with a partner, and rides her horse 4–5 hours a week (as well as making time for a psychotherapy practice!).

Benefits

There were more replies to the question, "What benefits do you derive from exercise?" than to any other question, suggesting that exercise serves a multipurpose positive function. These reported benefits can be broken down into the three general categories: physical effects, general emotional well-being and spirituality, and mental and cognitive effects.

Physical benefits included maintaining good health (feeling better physically); weight loss or maintenance of weight and healthy physical function (digestion, metabolism); increased strength, stamina, and muscle tone; improved sleep; and increased energy. One person commented, for example, "I don't currently train at the high intensity I did for gymnastics; now it's more for fun and health." Another has a chronic heart condition, controlled by medication, "but since I started this exercise regime, I have lost weight and feel stronger."

General emotional well-being and spirituality included stress relief, meditation, and calm; emotional release; and peacefulness. One person said that when exercising she "feel[s] more alive, more spiritually connected." Respondents frequently cited mental and cognitive effects, including cognitive clarity, a sense of control and a clearer head, self-esteem, and optimism. A prototypical global response was the comment, "I think it is an essential part of maintaining my self-esteem." Another person said, "When I exercise, I find that my mind gets clear of much of its clutter, allowing me to focus on issues and ideas." These responses corroborate the findings from McEntee and Halgin's survey of practitioner psychologists: "The amount a therapist exercises was related to how beneficial he or she feels exercise is to psychological functioning" (1996, p. 52).

Opportunities for socialization often are cited among the benefits of exercise involvement. Yet for this group who spend their days interacting with others, there was actually a bipolar distribution regarding the importance of social engagement. For some, exercise provided an opportunity for camaraderie and time to connect with others. For others, the separate time and space was a significant factor in their pleasure. Still others enjoyed forms of exercise, such as running, that allowed them the flexibility to be with others or alone. Combining many of these elements, one therapist described running 2 miles with her sister 5 days a week, and commented, additionally, "It gives me time away from my husband and my child."

Exercise Initiation and Maintenance

Therapists explained that they had begun exercising as a function of two influences, early modeling and adult health and physical concerns. Family modeling around activity in one's childhood, child and youth engagement in sports, and a general pleasure in physical fitness and the outdoors were mentioned by a number of people. Adult converts described concerns about health and illness, loss of muscle tone with aging, or weight concerns as initial motivators.

Beginning exercise and maintaining it are two very different experiences. When asked whether the reasons they had begun exercising were currently the same incentives, or whether other reasons had become more salient, general health and well-being were primary, even among those who have exercised competitively. One person commented, for example, "I wasn't aware of the emotional and spiritual benefits of exercise 16 years ago. I've become less obsessive about exercise and weight control." Overall, there was a sense that exercise has become incorporated into people's lives.

Thought Processes With Exercise

Because of my own personal experience of thinking differently when exercising, narrative responses seemed a means of finding out more about this real but nebulous area. Respondents were asked what they thought about when they exercise, and, further, whether there were qualitative differences between thinking while exercising and everyday thinking. I used examples from my own experience: I seem incapable of doing simple arithmetic when swimming; I have intense moments, during or shortly after exercise, of thinking more creatively. Some people commented that it is the opportunity to not think that is part of what makes exercise refreshing. Others described powerful shifts of thought. Some observed a sequence shift: initial mundane thinking that turned to body scanning or associative thinking (see Glossary), and then to the experience of pure sensation. Others portrayed a "free and released thinking." One person recounted deliberately using mindfulness meditation during exercise to lure out creativity. Some people noticed a trade-off: If they were training for competition, nonexercise-focused or dissociative thinking (see Glossary) was enough of a distractor to decrease the quality of the training.

EXERCISE RECOMMENDATIONS TO PSYCHOTHERAPY CLIENTS

Ninety-two percent of the female therapists and 96% of the male therapists responded that they recommend exercise to their clients. The frequency of such recommendations varied widely, however, from 10%–100%. Some focused on the goals achieved through exercise, rather than on exercise specifically. They recognized that these can be accomplished in a variety of ways. In part, practitioners' therapeutic orientation and style determined willingness to give advice of any sort. Some people did not see their role as that of making recommendations, although there was recognition that nonverbal office and interpersonal cues probably communicate their interest and engagement in activity anyway. One therapist who does not recommend exercise per se noted that the pleasure and value of exercise in her life are embedded in her "waiting room magazines, pictures, calendars, analogies, questions, vacations, working hours, and, occasionally, injuries."

Criteria for and Advantages of Recommending Exercise

Four general criteria for recommending exercise were articulated. Exercise is recommended as a means of coping with various clinical issues, specifically depression, anxiety, and overweight. Exercise is also suggested in order to cope with issues of daily living (i.e., improved sense of self, improved body image, and increased sense of internal locus of control and self-efficacy and mastery) through taking charge of one's own health, improving self-care, and decreasing passivity. Improved health and well-being and opportunities for increased social support were other reasons cited.

Although these reasons are similar, they are not identical to the reasons therapists gave for their own exercise. Appropriately, therapists' recommendations appeared driven by diagnostic and treatment concerns. It is interesting to note that the emphasis was more concrete (e.g., health) than abstract (e.g., thinking, spirituality). The mental benefits that many therapists themselves derive—and for which clients seek therapy—may not be at the forefront of therapists' attributions when considering the effects of exercise for clients.

Therapists described mixed success in the outcome of their exercise recommendation. Enthusiasm, resistance, and the opportunity to examine one's motives, goals, and actions were all mentioned.

Disadvantages of Recommending Exercise

Therapists reported a number of ways in which it might not be advantageous to recommend exercise. These included blows to the client's self-esteem, or a sense of shame, if they failed or perceived themselves failing in some way; a variety of interpersonal issues within the therapy itself, including transferential or countertransferential effects, or both; timing (i.e., recognizing that a client is not yet ready to implement an exercise regimen); and the potential for various negative physical effects of which the therapist might not be aware. One respondent summarized, "Some people just won't do it, they don't like it, aren't motivated, and feel badly about themselves reporting that they did not comply each week."

EXERCISING WITH CLIENTS DURING THERAPY

When asked whether they ever exercised with clients, the vast majority of therapists responded that they have not and would not. A few could imagine doing so and finding it helpful. Hypothetically, some people suggested that exercising with clients might allow a focus on the healing effects of exercise, increase the therapeutic bond, and be an opportunity to focus on motivational issues in a natural context. The stress reduction and health benefits for the therapist were noted, although this would be an obvious countertransferential hazard.

Three male therapists and three female therapists reported at least occasional exercise with clients during therapy. One psychologist, who works at a state hospital, commented, "Mild exercise is built into each morning's meeting, a procedure that I started. I also recommend 'gym time' for approximately 50% of the patients in the hospital that I am involved with. I have not found any disadvantages." Another, seeing outpatient clients, remarked that "they have to be receptive to it—and it must be productive therapeutically. They open up and become more relaxed and informal. Most are very receptive. Occasionally, clients get self-conscious or performance-oriented."

Many therapists noted a number of possible disadvantages or potential pitfalls to exercising with clients. The two primary concerns related to interpersonal boundaries and potential liability and malpractice issues. Additionally, concern was expressed that the ease of this elaborated dependency relationship might inhibit clients' risk taking in finding new exercise partners.

REFLECTIONS ON THE QUESTIONNAIRE RESULTS

The link between therapists' valuing of exercise for themselves and their support of the importance of exercise for their clients seems apparent. There may be some gender and age differences in therapists' own exercise experience. For example, women therapists who grew up in the pre-Title IX era may view exercise differently than their younger sisters. It is not clear whether there are therapist or gender issues (for the therapist or the client) in relation to recommending exercise to clients. It appears that exercise does not seem quite as foreign or "other" to male therapists as to female.

The mental and emotional benefits of exercise that therapists experience (e.g., problem solving, spirituality) can be highlighted when recommending exercise to clients and may help move the psychotherapy goals and agenda forward. Additionally, emphasizing the psychological benefits can draw clients' attention to this potentiality. Finally, because the psychological benefits point to meaningful and pleasurable aspects, these suggestions may increase the likelihood of exercise adherence as well.

Is a therapist's willingness to attend to the benefits of exercising with clients being overshadowed by the possible risks? We live in a time of increased awareness of the potential for boundary violation, compounded by an atmosphere of escalating litigiousness. An initial hesitancy to try a new process may be bolstered by these very real concerns. At the same time, is it possible to tease out these issues, in order to make use of this medium while diminishing the risks? The positive and perhaps synergistic experiences of those who have used this method suggest that too much caution may limit prospective opportunities. These questions and issues are addressed more directly in chapter 6.

Walking Through Working It Out

This book is designed to help therapists "work it out": to learn about ways in which exercise can be of assistance with a wide range of clients, from those acutely stressed to those with chronic distress, from youngsters to oldsters, primarily in the therapists' offices but occasionally out on the street. The physical benefits of exercise are well known. Here, the focus is on the mental and emotional benefits. *Working It Out* is intended to be read and understood by therapists who know therapy but do not necessarily know a tremendous amount about exercise, or sport. Its emphasis is exercise in therapy, although the literature and practice of sport psychology are valued as well. The primary focus is on clients. At the same time, this book also addresses—and may inspire—therapists themselves, to work out (i.e., exercise for themselves) and to work it out (i.e., expand their treatment focus and skills).

In section I, I delineate the basics of the body–mind connection. After giving essential definitions, in the first chapter I discuss the mental benefits of exercise and the ways in which exercise is a natural aspect of being human. In chapter 2, I present a matrix concerning the use of exercise in therapy, addressing client, therapist, and therapy itself. In chapter 3, I review a number of theories of therapy with regard to exercise inclusion, and invite therapists to begin a self-assessment of their use of exercise in therapy.

In section II, I address the specific manner in which exercise can be introduced into the therapeutic endeavor. In chapter 4, I explain the ways in which the transtheoretical model of change can be applied to participation in exercise. In chapter 5, I review the practical aspects of engaging clients in initiating and maintaining exercise. And in chapter 6, I provide a detailed description of the use of exercise during therapy, a relatively unexplored perspective. Although I acknowledge that this treatment method is one that will neither be appropriate for nor appeal to all clients or all therapists, it nonetheless seemed important to provide as much information as is currently available.

In section III, I examine the psychological benefits of exercise with a variety of populations—both clinical and demographic. I begin by focusing on those diagnostic categories for which adults most often seek outpatient psychotherapy. These are also the ones for which the greatest amount of research corroboration is available. In the latter chapters I consider exercise in relation to issues of psychological or medical recovery (trauma survivor empowerment and recovery from medical illnesses) and populations (diversity, life span, and athletes) across diagnoses.

In the final section IV, I offer a variety of necessary cautions in this work and support therapists in moving forward with practice development. Specifically, in chapter 18, I address the negative mental effects of exercise overuse, and in chapter 19, I address a variety of ethical issues of which therapists need to be aware. Chapter 20 is designed to help therapists with the next steps, and addresses education, training, and marketing possibilities.

A few points will help the reader work through this book more easily: Throughout, theory and research findings are illustrated with appropriately masked case descriptions. These vignettes are drawn primarily from my own practice, supplemented in a few instances by other therapists' experience. They are examples from real life, and I have deliberately included some in which not everything worked out perfectly. Without being confusing through this openness, I would like to convey my conviction that this fascinating method of practice is not simple and is not a panacea. Rather, it is complex and applicable in various ways to many people. It is this richness of possibility that is emphasized. At the end of each chapter in section III, I summarize and focus on the most salient points of use to therapists (Practitioner Recommendations).

The reader is invited to review the Glossary and Appendix A early and often. Especially for those unfamiliar with some of the terms routinely used in sport psychology (as well as, frequently, in cognitive–behavioral practice), the Glossary contains brief definitions of terms used particularly in the case descriptions. Appendix A, the Exercise and Sport Psychology Development Plan, is designed for practitioners to use as thoughts, ideas, and possibilities emerge during reading.

BASICS OF THE BODY—MIND CONNECTION

"Affective Beneficence": Exercise and Well-Being

1

The full complexity and intermingling of the relationship between movement and mind, or, in the language used here, exercise and therapy, cannot be summarized in a single word. Mindbody? Bodymind? Even German, that quintessentially words-strung-together language, can do no better than *leib-seele-einheit*, or body-mind-unity. The word *psychosomatic* carries with it an implication of pathology, the menacing and pejorative encroachment of a diseased mind on an innocent body. One possible descriptor is *behavioral physiology*, characterized as "the study of behavioral factors which result in organic changes from stress reactions" (Wiggins, 1996, p. 126). This definition, however, represents a unidirectional and rehabilitative focus. The novelty of another term, *somatopsychic* (Sime, 1996), allows us to reflect on the effects of physical action on our thoughts and feelings. It may be more descriptive of the multidirectional and interactive nature of effective exercise. Although none of these quite captures the nature of this holistic perspective, each can serve to remind us of the seamlessness of self.

Some years ago, Sime (1984) spoke of the exaltingly positive experience that can accompany or follow exercise. Targeting this sensation more specifically, Morgan (1985a) described exercise as having an affective beneficence. In this chapter I give an overview of that interaction. Before proceeding further, however, it is important to have common agreement about terminology.

Exercise, Sport, Therapists, and Clients: Initial Definitions

Along with appreciating the challenge of labeling this complex and interrelated undertaking, it is crucial when embarking on the dialogue between author and reader to share linguistic and conceptual understanding. Of relevance here is the language used to describe physical movement, practitioners, the people with whom we work, and the research and practice history from which we draw information for this work.

EXERCISE

Exercise is the term used throughout most of this book to mean organized, focused physical activity that involves a certain amount of exertion. It is distinguished from movement, which may be random. Except where indicated, exercise is also distinct from organized sports, in being noncompetitive. The term *sport*, or *sports*, is used here deliberately at times, recognizing that some clients are committed exercisers and are recreational or competitive athletes; that some athletes are involved in therapy; and that there are historical and continuing relationships between exercise and sport psychology.

The term *physical activity*, as compared with exercise, has been in ascendance over the past number of years (e.g., weight loss clinics prescribe "P.A."; current recommendations by the Surgeon General focus on the role of physical activity in people's lives rather than on sport per se; or the revision of a classic study on this topic: Morgan and Goldston's [1987] *Exercise and Mental Health* became, 10 years later, Morgan's [1997] *Physical Activity and Mental Health*). The advantage of the term physical activity is that it does not carry some of the pejorative obligation imputed to exercise. It could readily be interchanged with the term exercise as it is meant here. However, with half the syllables, the word exercise is an easier shorthand.

THERAPISTS AND THERAPY

The primary intended audience for this book is psychotherapists, or mental health practitioners, with training in such disciplines as psychology, psychiatry, clinical social work, mental health nursing, and marriage and family counseling. Emphasized here is the nature of the primary professional relationship, psychotherapy or counseling.

CLIENTS

For the most part, the people who are described here are those who are seen in outpatient psychotherapy. Mental health practitioners have debated the various merits of the terms *client* vs. *patient*. In general, the convention used here is to refer to the majority of people seen for outpatient therapy as clients. Those with more severe mental illnesses are described as patients.

EXERCISE AND SPORT PSYCHOLOGY

The primary focus of this book is the effect of the body on the mind through movement, labeled here as exercise, as an aspect of the psychotherapeutic armamentarium. Despite the definitional separation between exercise and sport mentioned above, separating out these concepts in interaction with psychology becomes more complex. Because of very different histories and implications, exercise psychology, sport psychology, and exercise and sport psychology each have different yet interrelated meanings. The effect of exercise on mental functioning is often considered one aspect of the field of sport psychology, forming, for example, the latter clause of the following standard definition. Sport psychology is "concerned with both the psychological factors that influence participation and performance in sport and exercise and the psychological effects derived from them" (Williams & Straub, 1998, p.1). In articulating the mind-body interaction, this definition highlights both those aspects generally referred to as sport psychology (psychological factors influencing sport) as well as exercise psychology (the influence of sport and exercise on psychological functioning). For a brief history of the organizational history of the field known most broadly as exercise and sport psychology, see Appendix B. Various terms commonly used in sport psychology, and referenced especially in case examples throughout the book, are described in the glossary.

Mens Sano in Corpore Sano: The Psychological Benefits of Exercise

A long legacy of either-or competition between mind and body has been evident in society, philosophy, science, and mental health. The body-mind dualism propounded by Plato, Galen, and Descartes is most evident in medicine in the biomedical model, "the view that all diseases and physical disorders are linked to disturbances in physiological processes" (Rejeski & Thompson, 1993, p. 7). Mental health practitioners often focus solely on the mind, viewing people in separate, competing, entities: mind and body. In doing so, therapists collude with clients in "cutting themselves off at the neck," thereby fractionating the self and missing some truly therapeutic opportunities.

A classical tradition of connection also has had its proponents. Best known is the phrase attributed to Homer, "*Mens sano in corpore sano*," a healthy mind in a healthy body. During the golden age of Greece, 24 centuries ago, much of the day involved vigorous physical activity, for children, adults, and the elderly. Deliberately, this activity was conducted for its contribution toward mental as well as physical well-being (Seraganian, 1993). And within psychotherapy, we have our own long history of recognition of this body-mind relationship. Freud conducted some of his analyses, including that of composer Gustav Mahler, while walking or hiking with his patients (Goode, 1998; Jones, 1967).

The biopsychosocial model that has emerged over the past 15 years reflects this current understanding of connection. This model takes "the position that the body, the mind, and the social context of human existence are reciprocally interdependent on one another" (Rejeski & Thompson, 1993, p. 7). As it supercedes the dualistic frame within medicine, the opportunity for new ways of understanding mental health and psychotherapy also can absorb this more complex understanding.

Renewed interest in health and well-being, albeit with decidedly mixed feelings and messages, has been the hallmark of the late 20th century. Numerous physical benefits of exercise have become widely acknowledged and accepted. Exercise, it is recognized, not only decreases coronary heart disease risk and improves rehabilitative potential, but it also impacts coronary risk factors, including high blood pressure, cholesterol level and type, smoking, and obesity. Exercise decreases the risk of colon cancer, and results in reduced body fat (or reduced total body mass and fat weight), lowered blood pressure, and improved carbohydrate metabolism. Exercise is associated with reduced problems or delay of problems related to diabetes, assists in the maintenance of bone density, helps improve the quality and quantity of sleep, and creates increased oxygen capacity. Overall, exercise is associated with improved health habits (Crandall, 1986; McDonald & Hodgdon, 1991; United States Department of Health and Human Services, 1996).

Less well known are the many psychological benefits. In a number of studies, exercise has been associated with decreases in depression and anxiety in both normal and clinical populations (e.g., Byrne

& Byrne, 1993; Kirkcaldy & Shephard, 1990; Klein et al., 1985; Morgan, 1985a; Raglin, 1990; Sime, 1984; Simons & Birkimer, 1988; Steptoe & Cox, 1988). Exercise also appears to have a positive effect on such psychological characteristics as self-concept, mastery, self-efficacy, self-sufficiency, body image, and cognitive processing (e.g., Berger & McInman, 1993; Ossip-Klein et al., 1989; Rodin, 1992; Sime & Sanstead, 1987). Seligman (1991) has noted the effects of optimism and pessimism on health status. The reverse, however, can also be true. Physical activity can affect people's positive valuing of the world. Exercise and sport can tap into and enhance one's sense of well-being, calmness, control, and attention to the present. Highly active people tend to be more optimistic and less pessimistic than those who are inactive (Kavussanu & McAuley, 1995). More mystically, moments of ecstasy, or a sense of awe and appreciation for the mystery of the universe, are sensations that can emerge from various activities (Csikszentmihalyi, 1990; Murphy & White, 1995).

> **I experience enjoyment and stress release. It's a combination of fresh air, enjoyment of the outdoors, strong sensory connection and fulfillment. Exercising in the outdoors gives me a full sensory and spiritual charge. Not surprisingly—to those who exercise regularly—I have more energy and am more alert, motivated, and focused when I have exercised regularly. Sunshine + light! are particularly important in the dark months and when all the daylight is during my work day.**
>
> **34-year-old female**
> **certified social worker**

Despite the apparent salubrious effects, therapists and clients live within social structures that, at best, give mixed and complex messages with regard to exercise. In the next section, I describe some of the conveyed societal messages that undergird a perception of exercise as obligatory. In contrast, I would suggest that a strong case can be made that exercise is a basic aspect of well-being.

Exercise as Obligatory vs. Natural

Increased media coverage of fitness issues and sports events, and a growth in the number of recreational facilities, would seem to reflect an increased recognition and acceptance of the benefits of physical activity. Yet, although attitudes may have shifted, the actual level and rate of physical activity has not increased. Exercise has been more popularized than popular (Berger, 1992; Brawley & Rodgers, 1993).

Reported increases in exercise may reflect expansion of physical activity among already active adults (Brawley & Rodgers, 1993). The greatest health benefit accrues when the least active become moderately active (Robison & Rogers, 1995), yet there is a dramatic decline in physical activity with age. Epidemiological studies show 65% participation between ages 10 and 17, but 15% between ages 18 and 64, and even lower rates thereafter. Lack of program adherence and dropout patterns are discouraging, although no worse than lack of adherence to programmatic change in relation to other health behaviors (Meichenbaum & Turk, 1987).

When exercise is viewed as obligatory, it becomes another chore. Instead, we can think of physical activity as central to being human. Dr. George Sheehan, dubbed the philosopher king of running by Bill Clinton, quoted another philosopher, Bertrand Russell, to bolster his argument about the pivotal nature of exercise to our being: "'Man is an animal, and his happiness depends on his physiology more than he likes to think. . . . Unhappy businessmen would increase their happiness more by walking six miles every day than by any conceivable change in philosophy'" (1996, p. 48).

As we have shifted from an agrarian economy to increasingly sedentary occupations, physical activity has disappeared from the daily landscape of our lives. In 1900, "almost all of us died of infectious acute diseases. . . . Today nearly all of us will die from chronic diseases. . . . Chronic diseases are not simply the *natural consequence of aging*. They appear, in large part, to be the consequence of an *unnatural lifestyle*" [*sic*] (Johnsgard, 1989, p. 16).

With increased leisure, exercise has become a task to be added to the day. As a culture, we have deluded ourselves into various beliefs about exercise.

We have decided that activity is effortful. In fact, activity begets energy. Using the Profile of Mood States (McNair, Lorr, & Droppleman, 1971), Morgan (e.g., 1985b) has consistently noted positive mood among active individuals and athletes. Morgan described the typical athlete mood pattern as an iceberg profile. With exercise, negative moods, labeled Tension, Depression, Anger, Fatigue, and Confusion diminish. Vigor, located at the center of the graphed score sheet, increases.

Our image of leisure time means *in*action: lolling on the beach, being transported on a carriage ride, or even the proverbial eating of bonbons while watching TV. The paralyzing, stultifying effect of (too much) leisure in some ways is comparable to the historical practice of binding upper-class Chinese women's feet. Rather than becoming freed to take pleasure in their leisure, their bodies were disfigured and their lives constricted by class and gender demands.

> I have a problem with the word "exercise." To me this connotes something I *should* do because it is *good for me*. "Recreation" or "play" or "fun" seems to capture more what I do and why.
>
> **49-year-old female psychologist**

If we think of activity as compulsory, it is neither fun nor pleasurable—when in fact, inherently, it is both. In an extended riff on the playfulness of exercise, Sheehan described three fundamental functions of play:

> Play is essential to the good life. We need it to become fully functioning human beings. . . . The first influence of play is on our bodies. It brings with it exercise. Medicine and surgery attack disease but they do not cover health. That resides in the fully functioning body, be it sick or well. Health is the best we can be. Health is getting the most out of the body we were born with. The playful use of the exercising body is what brings this about.
>
> The second influence of play is on our attitude. It encourages a sense of humor. . . . Humor allows us to be serious while having the feeling that it is all a game. Or we can come to a project knowing it is a game yet realizing how serious that game is.
>
> The final effect of play is on our conduct. . . . We must learn from ourselves. We must trust the inner person. The experiences in play are immediate, graphic, and illuminating. We learn the fundamental characteristics of our own personal human nature. In play we reveal ourselves—to others as well as to ourselves. Play is an unrivaled area for self-discovery. (1996, p. 62f.)

If activity is understood as unnatural and not part of everyday life, there is a concomitant sense that occasional or sporadic activity suffices. One has met one's obligation. The absurdity of this perspective can be understood by examining parallel assumptions regarding other natural aspects of being. For example, do we object to sleep at night? Do we plan to stock up on sleep so that we won't need to do it again? Do we say, "If I get 8 hours of sleep for 2 weeks, then I'll be perfectly rested for the next 3 months"?

These ridiculously rhetorical questions of course demand "No" for an answer. The same can be said for the necessity of movement. Being human involves meeting certain essential needs: eating, sleeping, and moving. "Regular exercise is required to fulfill our genetic design specifications for normal, trouble-free functioning" (Johnsgard, 1989, p. 23).

We remember Maslow best for developing the concept of self-actualization, the peak of his hierarchy of needs (1968). Maslow suggested that human beings function in an ascending order of needs. Certain needs (deficiency or D-needs) are so basic that unless they are met, there is not sufficient psychic or physical energy for the more esoteric (being or B-needs). In this sense, I am suggesting that exercise can be considered a D-need, essential to our experience of life.

Also relevant are Maslow's descriptions of both D and B aspects of various experiences, (i.e., D-love and B-love and D-cognitions and B-cognitions). From this perspective, exercise may be understood both as a D-state and as a B-state. It is both necessary and can be transforming. Although he did not elaborate on it, Maslow signalled his recognition of the multiple functions of exercise. One of the ways of being creative, a "raw, concrete, esthetic experience," is "(Greek style) athletics" (i.e., mind-and-body connecting; 1968, p. 209).

Pleasurable activity or exercise is, then, an essential component of our deficiency and being selves. Perhaps the greatest confirmation of this comes from how we feel—how we experience life—when we exercise. We are aware of a synergy that suggests this is how it feels to be optimally human. Our sense of well-being is increased. We experience a synchronicity and balance among the essential functions of being human: When we exercise, we sleep better, eat more healthfully, eliminate waste from our bodies more efficiently, and take more pleasure in sexuality. Descriptions of "peak experiences" or "the runner's high," although difficult to quantify, certainly underscore this view (Sachs, 1984c).

What is the connection between the pleasure, necessity, or value of exercise and therapy? What are some of the ways a therapist and client can explore these connections? I describe the relevance of these concepts to the psychotherapeutic endeavor in the next chapter.

The Client, Exercise, and the Therapist, 2

Even if one is convinced that exercise is essential to human being and that it can be experienced as pleasurable rather than compulsory, a connection between exercise and psychotherapy may not be immediately obvious; exercise and psychotherapy do not necessarily spring forth in the mind as natural bedfellows. The tool of exercise is the body, and that of psychotherapy, the mind. Yet these two apparently diverse areas can provide useful information to each other, as well as speak in concert. In this chapter I examine the ways in which exercise can be involved in psychotherapy.

The varieties of options available in psychotherapeutic exercise can be analyzed along three dimensions relating to the client, the therapist, and exercise. These are (a) the centrality of exercise or sport to the client's life and self-definition; (b) the degree to which exercise is involved in therapy; and (c) the role of the therapist in relation to the client and exercise. Within each dimension, engagement can range from none to extensive. Further, just as the process of therapy is not static, so these interactions are not unchanging. Although at any one time therapist and client will be in one particular point in regard to exercise, over time there may be shifts of engagement. Clients may become more or less physically active; issues around exercise may become more or less relevant to the therapy; and the therapist's role also may shift as exercise issues become more or less salient to the client. Further, some points along these dimensions cluster naturally together, whereas other aspects of the dimensions would not make logical sense. For example, recreational athletes may appreciate the therapeutic aspects of exercise and value therapists' modeling in relation to exercise. For physically inactive clients, however, the prescription of exercise as therapy could initially be experienced as irrelevant. These concepts are spelled out more clearly in the detailed descriptions that follow.

The Client's Level of Involvement in Exercise or Sport

How involved in exercise or sport is the client at the time that she or he is engaged in therapy? The importance of physical activity in the client's life will have direct bearing on exercise capability and salience. Indirectly, it also may relate to motivation. When examining the relationship of exercise and therapy, the therapist needs to assess the client's current exercise level.

Clients may vary along a continuum from physically inactive clients to professional athletes:

PHYSICALLY INACTIVE CLIENTS

These clients are sedentary. They do not currently exercise and may or may not recognize the physical and mental benefits of exercise. This group forms the vast majority of mental health clients. One of the goals of this book is to support the psychotherapist in assisting clients in becoming engaged in greater physical activity.

RECREATIONAL OR COMMITTED EXERCISERS

People may value or feel committed (Carmack & Martens, 1979) to regular exercise for various reasons. Typically, people are motivated by such factors as health, weight control, socialization, improved mental state, general well-being, or competition (Berger, 1984b; Sime & Sanstead, 1987). Clients are more likely to be physically inactive than to be recreational or committed exercisers. For these latter clients, however, more flexibility is possible regarding both the relationship of exercise to therapy and the therapist's role with exercise.

COMPETITIVE OR PROFESSIONAL ATHLETES

For these individuals, sport is a major source of livelihood or identity, or both. The therapist should be aware that athletes may be more averse than the general population to seeking help for their problems (Cogan & Petrie, 1996a), fearing that they will be perceived as deviant (Linder, Pillow, & Reno, 1989). Therapy issues that may be specific to athletes are addressed in chapter 17.

Competitive or professional athletes also may seek services for psychological skills training in regard to their sport (i.e., sport psychology as the term is popularly understood). A number of recent books will be of use to therapists interested in providing such services (e.g., Lesyk, 1998; Murphy, 1995; Van Raalte & Brewer, 1996).

Exercise and Therapy

When exercise is described as therapeutic or reference is made to exercise therapy, what is meant? Exercise can be therapeutic in that it is good for a person's well-being and relieves psychological distress. Rhythmic aerobic activities like running, brisk walking, cycling, or swimming have been the traditional forms measured when studying the relationship between exercise and well-being (Sachs, 1984b). More recently, Berger and colleagues (e.g., Berger & Owen, 1988,1992a) suggested that, at least among nonclinical samples, less strenuous forms of exercise such as hatha yoga might have similar positive effects on mood state.

In some situations, exercise itself is described as a central element or form of therapy. Further, exercise can be adjunctive to psychotherapy. In some instances, exercise becomes the medium in which the psychotherapy occurs.

EXERCISE THERAPY

Beyond its therapeutic nature, exercise has at times been prescribed as a type of therapy (Berger, 1984a; Brown, Ramirez, & Taub, 1978; Sachs & Buffone, 1984; Sacks & Sachs, 1981; Sime, 1984). In a now-classic study comparing running with verbal therapy for the relief of depression, Greist et al. (1979) pointed out that "depressive cognitions and affect seldom emerge during running, and when they do, they are virtually impossible to maintain" (p. 45). It has been suggested that through exercise clients have access to a variety of emotions, and "sports such as jogging are conducive to introspection as well as to thinking" (Berger & MacKenzie, 1981, p. 104).

Elevating exercise to the status of a specific form of therapy may have selectively important clinical utility. Exercise may function as the primary psychotherapeutic agent, especially in situations in which there is a biochemical aspect to clinical symptomatology. Some case examples illustrating this thesis are presented in chapter 7.

As is discussed further in chapter 18, exercise becomes neither therapeutic nor therapy when overused or used as a substitute for addressing real life issues (Raglin, 1990; Sachs & Pargman, 1984). Markers of exercise overuse include such cognitive and behavioral manifestations as increased depression, anger, fatigue, irritability, and a reduced sense of well-being (Morgan, Costill, Flynn, Raglin, & O'Connor, 1988).

EXERCISE AS ADJUNCTIVE TO PSYCHOTHERAPY

In general, a multimodal approach, in which exercise is encouraged in conjunction with psychotherapy, may offer greater success than either intervention used alone (Buffone, 1984a, 1984b; Sime & Sanstead, 1987; Summers & Wolstat, 1984). Support for clients' use of a combination of therapy and exercise is presented throughout the book. In section III, in particular, I highlight the therapeutic aspects of exercise with specific populations.

EXERCISE AS THE MEDIUM OF THE THERAPY

Popularized by Kostrubala (1977) at the peak of the running boom, exercise and verbal therapy conducted simultaneously has received only minimal anecdotal attention and no experimental research (Sachs & Buffone, 1984; Sacks & Sachs, 1981). Although the range of types of exercise may be somewhat limited (typically, walking or running), therapists who have used this method suggested markedly beneficial effects on mood, sense of well-being, and self-esteem (Hays, 1994b; Johnsgard,1989; Sime, 1996). This method is described more thoroughly in the next section of this chapter, regarding the therapist's role as participant in relation to the client and exercise. Further, information about and specific case examples of this method are described in detail in chapter 6.

The Role of the Therapist in Relation to the Client and Exercise

When supporting clients' use of exercise, what is the therapist's role? In one of very few explanations, Sachs (1982) defined *running therapy* as "the prescription of running as a mode of therapy" (p. 18). He then described the *running therapist* as "a psychologist, psychotherapist, or psychiatrist who uses running as a mode of therapy" (p. 20).

These definitions leave the practitioner with the question, still: What does the therapist do? How does the therapist stand in relation to the client? There can be a continuum of involvement by the therapist in the client's exercise. Minimally, the psychotherapist may be a consultant, or more actively, may serve as a role model. More interactively, during therapy the psychotherapist may be a participant with the client in the exercise.

When therapists become more active with their clients, whether verbally or physically, they must take care to understand and appreciate the various transference and countertransference implications of that increased involvement. Psychotherapy is a formal, hierarchical relationship that highlights and underscores such areas as power, authority, control, and the evocation of early emotional messages. By its very nature, issues including competition, achievement, and motivation are potentially and actually present in therapy. The specific expression of these issues varies according to the particular therapeutic dyad. Each of these may be exacerbated, clarified, or resolved when exercise becomes an element of therapy.

The more actively involved the therapist is with the client in regard to exercise, the more conscious she or he needs to be with regard to both process and ethics. These complex issues are discussed more fully in, respectively, chapters 6 and 19.

CONSULTANT

The psychotherapist who consults with a client about exercise may do so in a variety of ways. Among these are prescription, support and encouragement, or technical advice.

Prescription

In this role, the therapist suggests or encourages exercise as part of the treatment plan. Exercise may be designed specifically as a means to a treatment goal such as weight loss. Alternatively, the therapist may recommend exercise to ameliorate symptoms or conditions, such as in reducing anxiety or alleviating depression. This book is intended to assist the therapist in this role.

Obviously, the therapist needs some familiarity with, and information about, exercise. It is not necessary to know about all forms of exercise—a consultant, after all, is not a teacher. It is helpful, however, to be comfortable with some basic elements of an exercise prescription such as type, frequency, intensity, and duration. It also is important to have an awareness of available community resources.

Judicious use of one's knowledge precludes taking on dual roles. A psychotherapist also is not a coach. The psychotherapist has a unique opportunity to help create the best fit between a particular client and an appropriate type of exercise. Taking into account motivational issues, history of exercise, and such practical matters as convenience goes a long way toward ensuring the likelihood of adherence to an exercise regimen (Berger, 1984b). Appendix C offers therapists relevant areas to explore, including exercise history, behavior, decisions, and plans.

Support and Encouragement

As someone who supports and encourages the client to exercise, the therapist in this role appreciates the value of physical activity in the development of a sense of wellness or wholeness. Therapists who exercise, as well as those unfamiliar with particular forms of exercise, may take this specific stance. This role is especially useful when working with clients who already exercise—people for whom exercise forms one aspect of their lives or sense of self.

Technical Advice

Somewhat less prescriptive yet more directive, the therapist may function toward the client from more of an educational perspective. Especially with clients who are already exercising, the therapist may opt to offer technical advice with regard to mental issues and exercise or sport. For example,

- The therapist may teach the client specific mental techniques for performance enhancement, generically described as Psychological Skills Training (see Glossary).
- The therapist may give the client information about the interaction between psychological and physical factors such as the psychophysiological effects of exercise overuse (see chapter 18).

ROLE MODEL

Therapists who themselves exercise can be role models for their clients. They may disclose personal anecdotes about the benefits of exercise. They can provide or suggest resources to their clients. They have a natural authority or credibility when describing both the benefits and potential hazards of exercise, including the hazards of fanatical commitment.

It also is critical to recognize the role implications of gender. In our society, men and women are socialized about exercise and sports in markedly different ways (Birrell, 1988; Carlton, 1987; Rindskopf & Gratch, 1982). As a psychotherapist who exercises, I have been conscious that reference to my own exercising has at times resulted in invidious comparisons among female clients, whereas with male clients it has served to legitimize my stature and competence as a clinician. In chapter 6, I explore some of these dynamics in regard to interpersonal issues when engaging in exercise as part of therapy.

The following case description illustrates some of the role complexity that can occur in regard to the client and exercise:

> Fifty-year-old Brenda sought treatment shortly after she and her husband separated. A bright and capable woman, she was discursive, tearful, baffled about life, and approval seeking. She had a history of one previous hospitalization and was currently taking Prozac (20 mg. three times a day), as well as Xanax for sleep. She described herself, somewhat inconsistently, as a fitness instructor with hopes to run in a marathon in a few months. She was actually only running once a week, at some personal and logistical inconvenience.
>
> In our fourth session, in a discussion of various ways in which she could feel an increased connection to her internal and interpersonal life, I raised the question of running together during psychotherapy. Brenda's response was that she would not want to "impose." She said she would think it over, but the possibility was not discussed again, in part because of a foot injury she sustained, and in part because of an exacerbation of her problems that resulted in a brief prophylactic hospitalization.
>
> We terminated treatment a few months later. During the final session, for my own edification, I asked her about her earlier thoughts on running during therapy sessions. She described herself as having felt very uncomfortable. Because I was a sport psychologist, she *knew* that I ran farther, faster, and better than she. She had not wanted to inconvenience me. Although I had no objection to our not having run together, I regretted not having explored this decision earlier. Her assumptions about our running were a clear projection of many of her central issues: low self-esteem, the presumption that others are de facto more capable, and guilt, anxiety, and withdrawal if she did not accommodate to others' needs.

In some ways, Brenda's unwillingness to run during therapy had been a courageous act. Based on her beliefs, she had set some boundaries. Yet without discussion, the opportunity to underscore that aspect of her emerging definition of self also was lost. Dialogue around her decision might have been a useful and important means of examining and potentially resolving a number of issues apparent in other aspects of her life as well.

PARTICIPANT

Kostrubala (1984) advocated the use of exercise as part of the psychotherapy session. He noted that running therapy occurs outdoors, in a mobile and physically nonrestrictive setting. In contrast, the typical therapy hour takes place indoors, in a confined office. Despite his enthusiasm, Kostrubala recognized the power of the Pygmalion effect. Concerning the sources of the positive results he described, he cautioned: "My sample is too small to be of statistical significance, and I am unable to separate out the factor of my own enthusiasm which often affects the outcome of a treatment modality" (1977, p. 129).

Rindskopf and Gratch (1982) described a therapy program incorporating cardiovascular exercise (walking and running) and group psychotherapy with female clients. The 10-week sessions included a half hour of walking and running together outdoors, followed by an hour and a half of group psychotherapy. They found that the women then engaged in the group session with a sense of personal strength, energy, and accomplishment.

There is undoubtedly a synergistic impact when the therapist as a role model joins the client in exercise. Rindskopf and Gratch described how the shared activity can change the therapist's role:

> Participation is an equalizer; a strong power relationship becomes difficult to maintain. The therapist assumes the role of catalyst, of resource, and of partner with the client. Further, the onus of responsibility for change is placed on the shoulders of the client. . . . The locus of healing and eventually the locus for prevention are returned to the individual. (1982, 24f.)

Exercise as part of therapy is neither appropriate nor of interest to all clients. Although Sime acknowledged this reality, he nonetheless recommended that during initial counseling contact the therapist suggest that "it might be interesting and enjoyable to continue talking while going for a walk in the nearby vicinity" (1996, p. 175). Reflecting on the utility of exercise during therapy, he also commented (personal communication, February 11, 1998):

> A dramatic difference between exercise (walk-talk) therapy and traditional psychotherapy is that while walking side by side there is very little face-to-face conversation. This indirect interaction

may free up the client to be more spontaneous and thoughtful without regard to self-conscious concerns of appearance, behavior, and vocabulary. A client who might ordinarily feel uncomfortable in traditional psychotherapy tends to feel much more at ease or spontaneous in a discussion while walking simply because it has the appearance of being casual and unintimidating. Much like the exertional manifestations of deeper breathing and the more forceful expulsions of air in respiration, talking while walking elicits spontaneity.

Because the roles are shifted from those in traditional psychotherapy, therapists who conduct psychotherapy while exercising need to address a number of issues. Even more than the therapist who serves as role model, the therapist who exercises with a client at a minimum needs to examine questions of boundaries, intimacy, competition, dual role relationships, aggression, dependency, eroticization, and power. There are also potential issues of legal liability and confidentiality. To the extent that these areas are of concern, they must be dealt with as part of the agenda of the psychotherapy. Transference and counter-transference need especially careful monitoring. The therapist has a responsibility for addressing these issues in a thorough and ethical manner. In chapter 6, I address the complex and interesting opportunities afforded by exercising with clients during therapy. Ethical issues are considered there, as well as in chapter 19.

Putting the Matrix Together

Most clients seen by psychotherapists are physically inactive, people for whom exercise may be prescribed by the therapist as being therapeutic. Recreational exercisers, on the other hand, may appreciate the adjunctive value of exercise with their role model psychotherapists. Not all combinations of client, therapist, and exercise salience can logically exist. Physically inactive clients, for example, by definition would not use exercise as a form of therapy—until or unless they were to start being more active. Nonetheless, having these three dimensions to consider can increase the exercise-related options that therapists may review.

Does the use of exercise in therapy fit all therapies and all therapists? These dimensions are considered next.

Theory and Practice in the Therapeutics of Exercise | 3

Two powerful zeitgeist forces are heavily influencing mental health professionals as we enter the new millennium. The attention to holism (the body-mind connection described earlier) is one. The other is a life of practice that is in marked economic, business, and treatment flux.

Practitioners can respond to this latter tension through engagement with the energy of the former. Consultation and treatment approaches that address the entirety of being human, that allow for practice diversification, and that have versatility and flexibility, are especially valuable. Using exercise in therapy is such a method.

This chapter is designed to enable therapists to begin putting interest into practice. Both theory and practitioner are described. First, a number of theoretical frameworks are amenable to the addition of attention to exercise and sport psychology. Then, taking into account the practitioner's level of knowledge and skills as well as aspirations, I offer a method for self-assessment.

These topics are presented as if they were static and separate entities. However, it is in fact the specific mixture of theoretical understanding, practitioner interest and knowledge, and clientele that informs the unique practice. Although most of the book attends to exercise in therapy, at times exercise and sport psychology are seamless, interweaving with each other. This chapter recognizes and uses that reality. The case of Mike illustrates a number of the themes and topics that are elaborated throughout the rest of the chapter.

Responding to my Yellow Pages ad indicating "performance enhancement training for the athlete, performing artist, and business person," Mike, a 61-year-old business owner presented with three issues: an increased concern about mortality, the impact of fecal incontinence in relation to spastic colon, and negative mental scenarios in competitive golf situations. An impending prostate biopsy may have precipitated the contact. All the losses Mike had experienced and not processed— including the deaths of family members in an accident 25 years previously—seemed to be catching up with him. "There's a lot of death in this conversation," he noted in the first interview. His anxiety about incontinence meant that during daily 5 mi walks he spent considerable time anticipating and planning how to handle any emergencies. An avid golfer who saw physical activity as a way to counter mortality dread, his game was limited by catastrophizing thoughts and fears. He was clear that all of his concerns were related, and as treatment progressed, they wove together in synergistic ways.

Beginning with his presenting symptom, anxiety, I taught Mike various breathing techniques (see Glossary), to which he was immediately responsive. In session, he rated his level of tension as decreasing from a 5 to a 1 or 2 on a 10-point scale. Following the lead of his words, I also connected the calming breathing with a suggestion that he think "soft hands" as a cue word (see Glossary) as he gripped the golf club.

Following this session, Mike diligently practiced triangle breathing. He noted decreases in catastrophizing and general anxiety. Perhaps liberated by our discussion, he began speaking with others about some of his concerns.

Mike dropped out of and reentered treatment three times. In the process, we developed variants on relaxation training, and specific cues regarding his golf game. He learned that relaxation led to increased sphincter control. He felt supported in handling some aspects of prostate surgery. Although he valued the behavioral changes and their effects, he could never quite engage in tackling the deeper issues of loss, relationship, and life meaning.

Mike's initial choice of therapist was influenced by an appeal to two central aspects of his life: business and sports. And there was logic to this choice: His issues tangibly involved the mind and body interacting; he was responsive to techniques used in psychological skills training both in his everyday life and in relation to sports; and physical activity was a method used by him for symptom management. Responding to Mike in this manner with regard to these issues was an expansion of a prototypical therapy practice, rather than a radical departure. The underlying theoretical frames included a mix of cognitive-behavioral, psychodynamic, existential, and systems theories.

Reflecting on and evaluating one's practice is an ongoing endeavor. The inclusion of an exercise focus in therapy, and the perspectives and techniques of sport psychology, can be a dynamic addition to that process.

The Practitioner and Exercise and Sport Psychology

Filling nearly an entire wall of the Boston Museum of Fine Arts, a large and mysterious painting by Paul Gauguin titled "Where do we come from? What are we? Where are we going?" contains numerous figures of varying ages, seemingly in contemplation of their lives. The questions posed in the title of this painting are ones that reach into the deepest recesses of our beings. As well, they lie on the surface of our professional selves, as we assess what we have learned, what we know, and what we would like to be doing with our lives. Gauguin himself, of course, provides an interesting, if not exemplary, role model of practice evaluation and decision making: In his late 30s, he quit his day job as a Parisian stock broker and set out to be an artist in Tahiti.

As the case of Mike, above, exemplifies, it is the various mixes of being a therapist and a person knowledgeable about both exercise and sport psychology that are addressed here. Mike sought my services because the ad appealed to him professionally. Simultaneously cautious and suspicious of therapy and yet wanting relief from considerable anxiety and depression, he was able to make use of cognitive techniques within a sport psychology frame, receive support and encouragement for his physical activity, and apply mental techniques directly in his golf game. It also is important to acknowledge that the ways in which he circumscribed what he was willing to deal with and how he was willing to deal with it meant that some of the more profound aspects of his suffering could not be fully addressed.

Recently, Mehlenbeck, Coleman, Meyers, and Whelan (1997) surveyed members of the American Psychological Association's Division of Exercise and Sport Psychology (Division 47) and the Association for the Advancement of Applied Sport Psychology (AAASP) regarding actual sport psychology practice. Although respondents reported that they were engaged in sport psychology, the majority of these were people working in the sport sciences, in human movement or physical education departments of universities. Those in clinical or counseling psychology, whether university-based or practitioners, reported working an average of just over 10 hours a week in sport-related areas, with an average income of approximately $10,000 a year from sport-related work.

Although subject to all the limitations of surveys, these findings corroborate the general sense that I have had among practitioners with an interest in exercise and sport psychology. Even among those who have had considerable formal training in sport psychology, many psychologist colleagues are only working with a few pure sport psychology clients at any one time. This conclusion is certainly reflected in a pamphlet developed by Division 47 concerning graduate training and career opportunities in sport psychology (American Psychological Association [APA], 1994).

Rather than advocating for sport psychology practice per se, I would suggest that the already-established practitioner make use of his or her unique skills, talents, and interests and apply these to the general practice setting in regard to physical activity with clients. This premise forms the core of this book. Additionally, the practitioner may develop increased knowledge regarding performance enhancement training, the traditional purview of sport psychology.

Two overall components are involved in this practice development: the therapist's own theoretical framework for understanding and working with people, and her or his personal history and vision with regard to work in this field. Each of these areas is described below.

Theoretical Perspectives in Exercise and Sport Psychology

Which theoretical frames are effective in exercise and sport psychology? Although a quick perusal suggests a single perspective, in fact over the years a number of theories have been applied to working with clients, consultees, and athletes. Abraham Maslow suggested that if you have a hammer, everything looks like a nail. It is vital to understand the meaning of the particular hammer one is using, and to know which nails one is hitting, overlooking, or creating. One's rationale for intervention should be "coherent, logical, and theoretically and empirically well-grounded" (Cogan & Petrie, 1995, p. 283).

Therapists can maintain their theoretical perspectives and practice methods while adding knowledge and skills from exercise and sport psychology. The value of the hammer of one's already-known theoretical perspective is the therapist's sense of comfort and versatility with a particular approach. Rather than jettisoning these capacities entirely, various theories can continue to form the base of one's practice. Approaches that are less familiar to the therapist can be added gradually, as the therapist acquires the requisite understanding and skill.

COGNITIVE-BEHAVIORAL AND BEHAVIORAL METHODS

A Delphi poll suggested that the future of therapies lies in those that are brief, directive, present-centered, and problem-focused (Norcross, Alford, & DeMichele, 1992). In perhaps another zeitgeist phenomenon, sport psychology techniques have been developed and elaborated during the time frame that cognitive-behavioral methods have been ascendant within psychology and psychotherapy. Andersen and Williams-Rice (1996) commented that "much of sport psychology's repertoire of interventions comes directly from the cognitive-behavior therapy canon" (p. 282). In their concrete, direct, and educational focus, cognitive-behavioral methods also lend themselves well to psycho-educational applications performed by sport science-trained educational sport psychology consultants.

Perhaps most relevant, cognitive-behavioral methods tend to be effective. In a meta-analysis of cognitive-behavioral interventions among nonelite athletes, Meyers, Whelan, and Murphy (1995) reported an overall effect size of .62 for those receiving cognitive-behavioral interventions as compared with controls. Most of the current trade books on performance enhancement techniques focus on cognitive-behavioral interventions. These techniques comprise many of the methods described in the clinical cases in this book and defined in the Glossary.

Behavioral or rational-emotive methods also have been frequently used, for many of the same reasons. One of the first specific methods for working with athletes, for example, is a technique known as Visual Motor Behavioral Rehearsal (VMBR) (Suinn, 1986), combining relaxation training with cognitive restructuring and imagery training. Rational-Emotive Therapy, based on the work of Albert Ellis (e.g., 1994) and Reality Therapy, developed by William Glasser (e.g., 1976), also have formed the basis for sport psychology interventions (Acevedo, 1994; Martin & Thompson, 1995; Martin, Thompson, & McKnight, 1998). Others (Udry, 1992) have encouraged the use of Reality Therapy in supporting appropriate exercise behavior with clients.

PSYCHOANALYTIC AND PSYCHODYNAMIC THEORIES

Perhaps surprising to those whose interest in exercise and sport psychology has developed in the past decade or so, sport psychologists in the 1960s tended to approach the field from a personological perspective that often was rooted in psychodynamic theory. Considerable research was devoted to questions regarding the salient attributes of athletes' personalities (Cox, Qiu, & Liu, 1993). The depth of understanding and interpretation of meaning of sport is evident, for example, in Sacks' reflection that running provides "an adaptive response to losses that affect self-esteem and produce intrapsychic pain" (Sacks, 1981, p. 129).

> When I left my gym bag around in my office, I found that my patients began to carry gym bags and began to exercise.
>
> **52-year-old female psychoanalyst**

Because of its focus on the past, the unconscious, and healing, rather than the present, conscious thought, and education, psychoanalysis has over the years been attacked as irrelevant or even dangerous as both a theory of motivation and method of psychotherapy in the sport context (Gill, 1986; Martin, Thompson, & McKnight, 1998). Yet a wholesale rejection of psychoanalytic theory and practice can miss important internal and interactive dynamics. When clients do not engage in exercise, despite their good intentions, it may be that the pragmatic exigencies of everyday life are interfering. Additionally, or alternatively, therapists may find it significant and valuable to explore resistance and the transference process. The practitioner working with athletes may want to attend to both the adaptive and maladaptive aspects of defensive processes, transference, countertransference, and resistance (Seheult, 1997; Strean & Strean, 1998).

DEVELOPMENTAL COUNSELING PERSPECTIVES

Within sport psychology, a life span developmental model of counseling has been framed at times as an alternative to a more pathology-based clinical model. It focuses on the development of a sense of personal competence through the creation of goals, with concomitant strategies. The psychological skills developed in mental training programs often form the basis of focus within a more broadly defined application to life skill development for athletes (Danish, Petitpas, & Hale, 1995).

EASTERN AND EXPERIENTIAL PERSPECTIVES

Eastern philosophies, linking body and mind perhaps more smoothly than those of Western culture, have been used both as an approach to sport and in terms of the integrating function of the activities themselves. A series of books by Timothy Gallwey, originally written in the

1970s but recently revised and republished (1997, 1998), focuses on the "inner game," that is, the internal processing of activity in relation to specific sports. Gallwey posits an internal dialogue between two parts of oneself, the "teller" and the "doer." The goal is to diminish interference from the teller in order to optimize the potential of the doer. Physical skills are developed by means of mental skills, through observation, nonjudgmental awareness, creative images, and relaxed concentration.

> When I jog, the thinking is free and very creative. I come up with things I have 'no idea' where they came from. If I want a new idea about something or want to solve a problem, I'll bring my focus back to the topic, gently ask myself to think about it, and let my thoughts wander until I realize I'm off the topic, in which case I'll gently return my focus to the topic, or explode with some new idea.
>
> **42-year-old female psychologist**

A number of comparisons can be made between the *siddhi*, or Hindu power or capability, and sport experience or accomplishment. Murphy and White (1995) listed 29 parallel processes that have both psychological and physiological components. These ranged from the more pedestrian, such as exceptional control over mental and bodily processes, to the mystical, such as auras or out-of-body experiences. The Eastern Tao philosophy has been used both within sport and expanded to apply to all levels of one's life, including business and self-reflective development (Huang & Lynch, 1992).

In addition to philosophical understanding, various methods of meditation have been incorporated within action. Kabat-Zinn (1990) described "moving meditation" through slow, deliberative walking. Green (1995) has developed methods to combine running with meditative breathing. "Conscious breathing" while exercising, in which one "stays within one's breath," can increase stamina and improve concentration and focus, as well as allow for arousal regulation (Hendricks, 1995). Yoga and conscious breathing form both a therapeutic means and an end in and of themselves. My client, Barbara, for example, described more fully in chapter 16, began practicing yoga at age 74 in order to reinforce relaxed, deep breathing and decrease anxiety.

The various martial arts, such as judo, aikido, and karate, aim at integrating body and mind through symbolic as well as physical expression. The goal of judo, for instance, is "maximum efficient use of mind and body" (Gleser & Brown, 1988, p. 438). Gleser and Brown described using judo practice in therapy. Certain judo principles, such as yielding ("ju"), breaking balance, repetitive practice and rehearsal, also can have metaphoric meaning. And combinations are possible: Best known for his work as a cognitive-behavioral therapist, Wilson

(1996) used the analogy of karate and aikido to describe noncon-frontational methods of challenging obsessional and panicked thoughts.

In a similar vein, exercise has been used in Gestalt therapy to enhance focus on the present and explore symbolic meaning. Exercise can be used, for example, to underscore metaphoric activity, in contrast to passivity (Reynolds, 1996).

SYSTEMS THEORIES

The following case description involves an interaction of cognitive restructuring, Gestalt, and systems perspectives and methods.

Entering his senior year in high school, Carl, a 17-year-old football star, was determined not to do what he had done the previous two seasons: perform well when little was expected of him, but be filled with self-doubts, second guessing, and ineffective play when coaches began noticing his skill. In her phone call of referral, Carl's mother expressed concern not only about his sports performance, but also about Carl's increased irritability and general discouragement. She said, "He lacks vitality."

Carl, a large, sweet young man, was eager to be in treatment. He wanted to have a place where he could speak his increased self-doubts. "I lose belief in myself." A parallel theme emerged: A young woman he had dated for a year in a "difficult, consuming relationship" had recently broken up with him, with no explanation.

It was important to Carl to be able to deal with both his truths—in football and in relationships. And each interacted with the other. He experienced his self-doubts as huge. Using imagery, we focused on ways he might climb a metaphorical mountain of challenge. Easily, he recognized his athlete "self" as having the capacity to be strong, powerful, and elusive. As he wrote an "unsent letter" to his girlfriend, he was able to begin sorting out his own actions and the importance of letting the relationship evolve without his over-pressuring. In both instances, he was claiming his own self. As sport psychologist and clinician, I felt comfortable moving back and forth between sport performance and interpersonal relationship issues.

In the initial interview, Carl had described his own father's engagement in football, and the doubts he had experienced from *his* father, Carl's paternal grandfather, for whom "nothing was good enough." For the third session, Carl was intrigued to have his father join us, in order to better understand the intermixed messages within the family around sport, achievement, and masculinity. In session, Carl's father was forthcoming about his own adolescence, perfectionism, paralyzing fear, and self-denigration. Although Carl had had some general sense of his father's developmental experience, these specific stories and concerns came as a revelation to him. Not only did he come to know about his father's reality, he was enthralled at the mirroring of much of his own feeling.

The openness of this session was healing for both participants. I could sense myself speaking to each of their needs in suggesting true internal acceptance, in contradistinction to the paternal grandfather's competitiveness. Father and son could incorporate their deeper appreciation of each other into their sense of self.

There are a number of ways in which a systems perspective may have relevance to exercise and sport. Among these are the prescription of exercise within families (e.g., Epstein, 1992), working with families of athletes, and an awareness of the context (system) within which athletes perform.

Sport psychologists have described the interrelation of actual family and athlete (e.g., Coppel, 1998; Hays, 1998; Hellstedt, 1995; Stainback & LaMarche, 1998). Concepts from family systems theory, including differentiated cohesion, triangulation, resistance, effective communication patterns, and hierarchy, also can be applied to work with sports teams (Brown, 1998; Oglesby & Hill, 1990; Zimmerman, Protinsky, & Zimmerman, 1994). The athletic subculture, athletic identity, social networks, and leadership characteristics are areas that readily lend themselves to a systems perspective. Issues around athlete academic performance, overtraining and burnout, and unhealthy weight control practices all are affected by intragroup beliefs and practices (Brustad & Ritter-Taylor, 1997).

Many sport psychology interventions focus on the individual athlete, and educational sport psychology methods are often presented to an entire team as if they were one. A contextual and systemic focus, however, is frequently of importance both in conceptualizing interactions and in delivering services. Carr and Murphy (1995) extrapolated the four general functions of the family system to team functioning, within a "team-as-family" dynamic: establishing the system's general attitudes, expectations, values, and goals; issues of power and authority; management of change; and patterns of communication.

The perspective of community psychology, with emphasis on context, prevention, and relational community, has been explored on occasion (e.g., Hays, 1992; Lamont-Mills & Pretty, 1997). In their consultation program with female collegiate gymnasts, for example, Cogan and Petrie (1995) developed an intervention based in part on the specific cohesion characteristics of this particular sport.

FEMINISM

Although feminism is not theory-specific with regard to practice, certain principles underly feminist practice, relating to social systems and the politics of gender. Feminist theory recognizes the sociopolitical, cultural, life span developmental, and historical context. It uses an empirical base, derived from interdisciplinary study, and grounds experience in women's lives. Especially attentive to issues of power, exploitation, and misogyny, feminist practice focuses on strengths more than deficits, and is action focused. A feminist perspective can address issues around the social and contextual issues of engaging women in exercise (Hays, 1994a). Likewise, many sport-related issues have a socially engendered component, including body image, eating disorders among athletes, the uses of aggression, sexual harassment in sport, or homophobia and compulsory heterosexism (Duquin, 1994; Gill, 1995; Nelson, 1994). The potential to rethink sport or exercise engagement from the perspective of relational theories offers many new avenues for men as well as women (Bredemeier et al., 1991; Oglesby & Hill, 1993; Wildman, 1998).

OTHER PERSPECTIVES

A technique rather than a specific philosophy or theory of therapy, hypnosis has been linked to exercise in various ways. A Hungarian method described as active-alert hypnosis uses stationary bicycle pedaling to induce hypnosis among clinical patients (Bányai, Zseni, & Túry, 1993). Hypnosis also has been used for many years as a treatment method with athletes (Morgan, 1993).

The use of physical movement in therapeutic recreation or dance and its connection to physical education has been recognized through structural links within physical education departments and professional groups (e.g., the American Alliance for Health, Physical Education, Recreation and Dance [AAHPERD]). Although occasional connections have been made (e.g., Menapace & Stern, 1998; Serlin & Stern, 1998), there are only limited references in the sport psychology literature to somatic methods, such as Feldenkrais or Functional Integration. Despite the considerable overlap with the various body therapies, there has been little integration in applied sport psychology.

On a sport psychology electronic mail list, recent postings suggested that some practitioners are applying a variety of clinically developed techniques, such as Neuro-Linguistic Programming, and some newer approaches, including the "power therapies," such as Thought Field Therapy. The effectiveness of these methods has not been established, and there are many concerns around appropriate training and underlying theory. Additionally, it is not clear whether methods developed to assist in resolving trauma have applicability to situations that are normative. A few case studies of the use of Eye Movement Desensitization and Reprocessing (EMDR) have been described at recent sport psychology conferences and in the literature (Foster, 1997; Lendl, 1997; North, 1997; Oglesby, 1995; Wildenhaus, 1997).

Although a body of literature has not yet developed around their use with athletes, other theoretical perspectives and psychological techniques have been described by some practitioners. For example, the eclecticism available within exercise and sport psychology is evidenced by pairing Reality Therapy with a method developed within community psychology 30 years ago, Goal Attainment Scaling (Martin & Thompson, 1995). Narrative therapy has been used in working with a women's rowing team, to clarify individual and group relationships and support team functioning within the social context (Schmelzer, 1996). The prescription of exercise would seem a natural option within the pragmatism of solution-focused therapy (O'Hanlon & Weiner-Davis, 1989), for example with regard to individual or team goal setting (Wildenhaus, 1997).

The Exercise and Sport Psychology Development Plan

Information concerning practice development and marketing is presented in the final chapter of this book, yet the reader is encouraged to read in an active and interactive manner. Whether it be vignette, research findings, or practice recommendations, it is hoped that much of the material will spark an interest and have relevance for one's own practice. To capitalize on that process, the reader is encouraged to make use of Appendix A, *The Exercise and Sport Psychology Development Plan*, while reading this book. The reader's history, current practice, and intentions are each and all relevant to sections on self-assessment, professional issues, office issues, financial plan, and marketing. The development matrix is designed to help the practitioner focus on the most relevant populations and issues, categorized in terms of skills and knowledge one already has, skills and knowledge one needs to develop, and areas that are of especially high interest for one.

Certain key elements inform the adventure of practice development, whether one is looking at current practice or plans. Past history, current life, and future intentions—Gauguin's questions—all affect one's planning.

WHERE DO WE COME FROM? PERSPECTIVE AND HISTORY

When reviewing one's own history as background for this type of work, certain features may be relevant:

Physical Activity History

Recognition of and appreciation for the importance of exercise in well-being frequently derives from therapists' history of physical activity, which may or may not have been in a competitive sport setting.

History as a competitive athlete often is a prelude to interest in exercise and sport psychology. Not surprisingly, often people are drawn to the particular sport that they played. Although in general this history nurtures motivation, there is a potential for complications of overidentification (Yambor, 1997; Yambor & Connelly, 1991).

Coaching History

Similarly, coaching often draws people toward exercise and sport psychology. As with one's history as a competitive athlete, this history can potentially have benefits and drawbacks. Along with the advantages of knowing the sport and its practice from a particular vantage point, issues of role diffusion (Ellickson & Brown, 1990) and overidentification (Yambor, 1997; Yambor & Connelly, 1991) need to be recognized.

Other Performance History (Dance, Music, Acting, etc.)

The mental aspects of effective performance, such as arousal regulation, goal setting, and imagery, have some universality across performance domains. Thus, a history of engagement in the performing arts can be of considerable utility. Additionally, this perspective can assist the practitioner in broadening his or her range of practice. At the same time, lack of familiarity with the sport setting and with sport science can limit some of what one brings to the field.

WHAT ARE WE? PRESENT ACTIVITY

The practitioner who values general well-being and has a holistic perspective is in a good position to adapt the information provided in this book to his or her own practice. Whether within the competitive realm or not, a history of or present involvement in physical activity helps give one an appreciation for the concrete ways in which mind and body work together. It also can add legitimacy to the therapist's self-presentation. Messages regarding client self-care are received as more valid when presented by a healthy and fit practitioner.

WHERE ARE WE GOING?
PLANS AND INTENTIONS

Thinking forward, toward who one would like to become, is a process of discovery and clarification. By analogy, one can think of an investigative reporter, asking the five Ws + 1. Broadly defined, these questions include:

Who do you want to work with? What kinds of clients do you see now, and how is that similar to or different from who you would like to be working with? This forms the "row" portion of the development matrix in Appendix A.

What do you want to do? Is the focus primarily one of assisting clients (a general or specific population) to exercise as part of their therapy? Is it, rather, working with athletes regarding performance enhancement? Responses to these kinds of questions form the basis of the "columns" portion of the development matrix in Appendix A.

Why do you want to do it? Broadly speaking, what will you get out of this type of work? People often think of this aspect in terms of both intrinsic and extrinsic goals.

When do you want to do it? This question speaks to one's sense of commitment to and focus on this type of practice, whether it is one's entire caseload, part-time specialization, or blended within one's work.

Where do you want to do it? One of the determinants of exercise and sport psychology practice relates to setting and location. Seeing clients in one's office is different from workshops offered at a health club, and, in turn, differs from working with a university sports team.

How do you want to do it? An assessment of one's current skills as compared with one's aspirations points to the steps necessary to get from one to the other. The circles, squares, and triangles within the development matrix are useful ways to visualize responses to this question.

In the next section I move from theory toward practice. The client is in the foreground as discussion focuses on the engagement of clients in exercise within the context of therapy.

II | CHOOSING EXERCISE AS A THERAPEUTIC TOOL

The Process of Change | 4

H aving established the value of exercise for mental as well as physical well-being, in the chapters in this section I focus on ways in which therapists can work with clients in the development and maintenance of exercise. This is a natural process for therapists: The therapeutic milieu involves change; exercise and psychotherapy can have complementary functions; and psychotherapists focus on individual assessment, prescription, and evaluation.

Therapists see people at a time when their lives are in flux. Crisis theory suggests that at times of crisis people may be most amenable to change. Therapists are, above all else, change agents. The therapist is in an ideal position, then, to assist the client not only in assessing issues, but also in developing new coping methods.

The combination of exercise and therapy, addressing both physiological and cognitive processes and their interactions, may be more powerful than either alone (Buffone, 1984c; North, McCullagh, & Tran, 1990; Sime & Sanstead, 1987). One implication is that this multimodal treatment may result in more effective and efficient use of therapy. Potentially, clients who engage in both psychotherapy and exercise may make better and more rapid use of psychotherapy.

Mental health practitioners can play a number of important, even pivotal, roles in this process. They may assess clients' readiness for exercise. They may help clients develop individually appropriate exercise patterns. They may monitor both short- and long-term exercise benefits in regard to mood or other symptoms. Therapists also can assist in exercise maintenance.

In this chapter I review a theory of motivation that can be usefully applied to exercise. Following that, in the next chapter I focus on the specific factors relevant to helping clients begin and continue exercising. In the third chapter in this section I present some case studies of the use of exercise incorporated into psychotherapy.

Stages of Change

Of particular use in assessing clients' readiness for the development of new behaviors is the "transtheoretical model of behavior change," often referred to as Stage Theory. It was developed originally by Prochaska and DiClemente and has since been elaborated in conjunction with other colleagues. (See Prochaska, Norcross, & DiClemente, 1994 for a popular version of this theory, easily comprehensible to a lay audience.) They focused on a number of health behaviors, including smoking cessation, alcohol use, mammography, and weight reduction. The transtheoretical model contains three assumptions about change: (a) change involves much more than an all-or-nothing or on-off action; (b) at any time people are in one or another stage of change; and (c) specific interventions are more or less relevant at different stages. The model is described as transtheoretical because techniques applicable to various therapeutic modalities—psychodynamic, cognitive, and behavioral—are appropriate interventions at different stages of change.

If one thinks of human beings as engaged in some aspects of change at all times in their lives, the broad sweep of this model becomes apparent. The interested reader, for example, could assess their own stage with regard to "readiness to encourage clients to use exercise to improve their health and sense of well-being."

In the past number of years, Marcus and others have applied this model to the adoption and maintenance of exercise behavior. The stages, as they may be applied to exercise or sport (Marcus, Rakowski, & Rossi, 1992), are:

> Precontemplation: "I currently do not exercise and I do not intend to start exercising in the next 6 months";
> Contemplation: "I currently do not exercise, but I am thinking about starting to exercise in the next 6 months";
> Preparation: "I currently exercise some, but not regularly";
> Action: "I currently exercise regularly but I have only begun doing so within the last 6 months";

Maintenance: "I currently exercise regularly and have done so for longer than 6 months."

Some aspects of this model are especially captivating. For one thing, this framework can be used to describe almost any change, whether one is talking about actual behavior or thoughts and feelings. Thus, for example, the client who mentions seeing a recent report on exercise and health may be indicating a shift in attitude preparatory to actual behavior change.

Furthermore, the model co-opts all of us: You cannot not be in one of the stages. Ergo, you are in the process of change. Finally, the model is entirely grounded in the human experience. In fact, I often describe these concepts to clients in the following manner:

> Sometimes we think that change is like an on-off switch. First you weren't doing something, then you decided to change and voilà! you began doing it. For example, you may assume that losing weight is just a matter of will power, of deciding to go on a diet and lose those extra 10 pounds. In fact this theory suggests that that's the fourth stage of change, and it's called the action stage. But people are much more complicated than the either-or model suggests. Change is a process. It takes conscious effort to shift long-standing habits. Before you're ready to take action, you may spend quite a while thinking about it, trying it out, and kind of going back and forth. In terms of weight loss, you may go on a drastic diet for a few days. Or, you may stock up on healthy foods that you like. That's stage three, the preparation stage. Before that, there's even more thinking, as you contemplate even taking the action. You probably would be really alert to media stories about life-style changes, or appropriate BMI (body-mass index) ratings. You may think about other times you've attempted to lose weight and begin sorting out what was useful. But there's even a point before contemplation, which is called precontemplation: Other people around you may think you should do something, but you aren't even considering it. This time of rationalizing and discounting can take many forms: "I'm under too much stress"; "It's good to have some extra padding in winter, and so on."
>
> There's also stage five, because once you do change, it takes a while for it to become a habit. So the fifth stage is maintenance, which may be the most challenging stage of all. People who lose weight and are able to maintain that weight loss typically find that there is a whole range of life-style changes that accompany this process, and it takes time and repetition to truly understand and make use of those alterations.

Across 12 behaviors, a general pattern of stages has been noted: 40% of people are in precontemplation, 40% are in contemplation or preparation, and about 20% are in action or maintenance (Prochaska, 1996; Prochaska & Marcus, 1994). Since the likelihood of changing behavior doubles with each change of stage, an appropriate (and morale-enhancing) goal for both therapist and client may be to assist a client to progress one stage in the next 6 months (Prochaska, 1996).

The stages of change are affected by a number of processes by which people change their behavior (Prochaska & Marcus, 1994). These processes can be clustered into experiential and behavioral constructs. The experiential processes involve information gathering, affective issues, and reappraisal of one's values and impact on others. Behavioral processes include counterconditioning, helping relationships, reinforcement management, and stimulus control. Experiential processes are typically of more value in the early stages of change, whereas the behavioral processes appear to be more central to the latter stages. Although this distinction has proved accurate in various studies of smoking cessation, in a cross-sectional study of exercise adoption and maintenance among a large community worksite sample, participants tended to use the experiential as well as the behavioral processes well into the action stage (Marcus, Rossi, Selby, Niaura, & Abrams, 1992). Thus, respondents already exercising continued to find it important to take stock of their behavior (self-reevaluation) and reflect on its importance to others (environmental reevaluation), for example, processes that for other kinds of behavior change are generally important during contemplation. This may reflect the need for multiple determinants and supports in developing a pattern of exercise as a regular and continuous aspect of one's life.

PRECONTEMPLATION

People tend to be in the precontemplation stage with regard to behavior change for a number of reasons. They may be uninformed about the long-term effects of their behavior, or demoralized and unwilling to think about this behavior, or defensive about changing. Perhaps they recall how much they hated or felt humiliated during high school physical education classes, and think that exercise now will feel the same. Or they may have tried exercise a few years ago but fell off the wagon. Although there are more than 50 benefits from 60 min of exercise, precontemplators are able to come up with only five or six benefits (Prochaska, 1996).

To assist a client in moving from precontemplation to contemplation, various "experiential" methods that increase people's awareness of the salience of exercise are relevant. Reflective therapy is especially helpful during the precontemplation stage. The therapist can help the client identify and begin addressing defenses. Denial, rationalization, and intellectualization are among the most obvious ways clients tend to maintain the status quo. In this stage, the client may be receptive, even if not responsive, to information. For example, many clients are entirely unaware that exercise may have mental as well as physical benefits.

> Carrie, age 40, seemed an ideal candidate for the beneficial effects of exercise. She was depressed, overweight, and expressed motivation to change. Although she had a history of severe and chronic physical illness, she was now in adequate physical condition and being carefully monitored by her physician. She knew that she should exercise, and she occasionally went for a walk. This seemed the most likely form of exercise, and we worked on environmental issues (time of day, frequency, duration). While appearing responsive, in fact Carrie did not follow through. Over time, it became apparent that she had a pattern of sweetly not complying with expectations. Her passive resistant style in regard to exercise initiation reflected a stance that maintained dependency and hesitancy about "ownership" of herself. Discussion about this style needed to precede any movement toward exercise, although the issue of exercise, and more broadly, self-care, could become a measuring ground for change.

CONTEMPLATION

Contemplation is a fascinating stage, a space that clients may land in or return to quite often. It is the high point of ambivalence. In this stage, a key issue involves helping clients become emotionally and cognitively engaged in the process of change. It is the moment to develop a "decisional balance scale" of the benefits and costs of exercising. The client can assess both the pros and cons of the contemplated behavior change, in terms of consequences to and reactions of oneself and others. (See Appendix C for an example of a Decisional Balance Scale.)

> Exercise was such a stumbling block for me that I wrote my dissertation on the subject. Over 2 years I have finally made a longlasting significant change in my eating and exercise habits, but I stayed in contemplation for a very, very long time.
>
> **32-year-old female psychologist**

One of the biggest mistakes in beginning exercise is to spend too little time in contemplation and preparation, leaping into action, relapsing, and feeling confirmed in one's belief that one is a failure. Encouraging contemplators to action too vigorously can result in resistance and a retreat to precontemplation (Prochaska & Marcus, 1994). On the other hand, self-efficacy for exercise, one's belief that one is going to be successful in this process, is a key developmental aspect of the contemplation stage (Prochaska & Marcus, 1994).

> Trying to help a client take action when s/he is really in a contemplation stage can lead to lower self-efficacy.
>
> **32-year-old female psychologist**

Dependent and depressed, 48-year-old Joan was sinking into a deeper and deeper emotional hole at the point where she truly began contemplating exercise. She recognized that inactivity increased her depression and her sense of helplessness. She sought out the support of others in considering undertaking this change of activity and self-view. She recalled her sense of well-being and the pleasure she had taken when she had exercised for a few months. We discussed the anticipated impact (positive and negative) her exercising might have not only on herself but also on her family. She developed an increased sense that this time, with her thoughtful planning, she would be able to create an exercise pattern that she might be able to sustain.

PREPARATION

Making a commitment to change is the hallmark of the preparation stage, and with that can come considerable anxiety, ambivalence, and self-doubt. Reworking the decisional balance scale to increase the number of pros vs. cons for exercise can be helpful. Doubling the list of pros results in a stage change (Prochaska, 1996). Helping a client own her process of change is especially critical at this point. The therapist may reflect with the client on attitudinal changes that have already occurred, or review with the client his automatic thoughts and rational responses after he has attended a road race. The therapist may listen carefully for the client's readiness to set a start date for exercise.

As the following case illustrates, early focus on the practical aspects of exercise can lead to a classic transactional analysis game of "why don't you—yes but" (Berne, 1964). Later attention to these issues was perceived as supportive of the client's increased autonomy and skill in self-care.

> Having tried a number of commercial weight loss programs, Sara entered therapy feeling discouraged about herself, her life, and her parenting skills. She was also still reeling from the effects of a long-term abusive marriage that had ended 3 years ago.
>
> At one point during the marriage, she had run on a daily basis. Now, however, she felt uncomfortable about being outside, alone, for a period of time. She feared that her ex-husband might stalk her. Instead of focusing on weight, self-image, and exercise, therapy centered initially on finding genuine ways she could experience power with regard to basic life issues: at work and in regard to continuing concerns about custody of her children.
>
> As she began to feel competent in work and parenting, Sara was willing once again to tackle the question of her body image.

She tried out various extreme diets before settling into a nondeprivation method of eating control. Although she was aware that exercise would assist in weight loss, in the past she had used exercise to cheat on diets (i.e., exercising to balance overeating). She decided to postpone regular exercise until she felt committed to the weight loss program she had designed for herself. When she was ready, she bought a treadmill and used some parts of therapy sessions to figure out the logistics—when she would use it, where to place it so that she would actually use it, how to build up her use gradually. A weekly graph of weight loss and exercise helped her see change over the long term and reinforced her sense of competence.

ACTION

Action is the stage at which overt behavioral change has taken place with some consistency. It also is the stage with the highest risk of relapse. The important interventions here tend to be those that are behavioral. At the same time, this is the stage in which the greatest number of change processes are used (Prochaska & Marcus, 1994). Keeping track of what one is doing, what the actual obstacles are, and ways in which the environment can support this change are all critical components of this stage.

Norman began exercising almost as soon as it was suggested to him. A gangly and disheveled 53-year-old middle manager, he had been caught off guard by a major depression serious enough that in pre-managed care days he would have been hospitalized. This episode of depression had begun some 3 months prior and not been successfully treated with Zoloft. "It appeared to help for one and a half months and then I felt like I fell off a cliff," he reflected. Already gaunt, Norman reported insomnia, lack of appetite, problems with concentration, severe self-doubt, and uncontrollable emotional lability and tearfulness. He was referred for therapy by his physician, who had recently started him on Serzone (150 mg. b.i.d.).

Norman reported one other instance of severe depression, 30 years prior. Although there were some significant recent losses that might be precipitants of the current depression, endogenous factors seemed paramount. Assuming that treatments affecting biochemical balances may be helpful, one of my first suggestions to him was to begin aerobic exercise.

Slowly, and without much satisfaction, Norman began riding his bicycle for 20 minutes a day. His lack of pleasure indicated that the bicycle riding might not be having an antidepressant effect. Further, given the combination of his depressed state and this lack of positive effect, he was likely to discontinue exercise. I asked if there were other kinds of exercise he had enjoyed in the past. His face lit up as he described roller skating. Since there was no rink less than an hour away, we discussed the possibility of in-line skating. Shortly thereafter, he bought skates, and rapidly worked up to skating three to four times a week for about 45 minutes at a time, often using this as his mode of transportation to and from work.

Some months later, we again reviewed Norman's exercise behaviors and plans. As autumn approached and Norman became concerned about the possibility of a seasonal component to his depression, he wanted to plan exercise that he would be able to do through the winter. Ice skating or aerobic classes seemed promising options.

Norman's depression gradually remitted. In my judgment, the significant factors, in order of importance, were medication, exercise, and psychotherapy.

MAINTENANCE

Maintenance involves processes similar to the action stage, focusing on those processes that reinforce the maintenance of behavior change. Two factors are central to maintaining the changed behavior over time: sustained, long-term effort and revision of one's life-style. Social pressures, internal challenges, and special or atypical situations are factors most likely to undo the changes that have been made. To maintain new exercise behaviors, it is especially important to support and find supports for one's positive beliefs and to avoid overconfidence. Overconfidence can be a way to court relapse, since it involves a lack of mindfulness to important supports and warning signs, and an overreliance on one's willpower to sustain change (Marcus, Rossi, et al., 1992; Prochaska, Norcross, & DiClemente, 1994).

Predicting and developing strategies for handling lapses prevents them from becoming relapses.

> 26-year-old Kris, described more thoroughly in chapter 13, entered therapy with specific body image issues and mild anxiety and depression. Because she and her husband were considering pregnancy, she was unwilling to use psychotropic medication for the depression. She had begun regular walking just prior to the start of therapy.
>
> Throughout therapy, we discussed exercise as one part of her evolving sense of self. Kris began to work out on a friend's equipment for a while, then joined a health facility and made time to go there regularly.
>
> Kris responded well to therapy, gradually tapering visits. As therapy drew to a close, 8 months later, Kris had taken a new job in another state, and her husband's occupation allowed him to move without difficulty. Among the first aspects of the new environment that Kris and her husband assessed—along with housing options—were available health facilities.

RELAPSE

"No matter what we do, the majority of people will relapse after any single attempt to overcome most chronic behavior problems" (Prochaska & Marcus, 1994, p. 168). Numerous studies report that 50% of people embarking on exercise programs do not continue them for more than 6 months (Dishman, 1988). Findings from various programs designed to decrease negative behaviors, such as smoking cessation, suggest that people cycle through the stages of change many times before finally ceasing the undesired behavior. Positive life-style changes may likewise need a number of iterations before becoming permanent. It is helpful for the person who has relapsed to assess: What did I do right? What mistakes did I make? What were the "trigger events" (e.g., stressful thoughts or situations) that preceded the relapse? What do I need to do differently next time? (Gorski, 1989; Prochaska, 1996).

> Alice, described more completely in chapter 6, began exercising for weight loss, affect control (anger and sadness), and anxiety management. After 6 months of walking or riding her bicycle on a daily basis, she felt entirely committed to exercise as part of her definition of self, paying continuous and careful attention to the ways in which exercise served to help moderate her mood and stress. A combination of revised eating behaviors, social support, psychotherapeutic insight, and exercise resulted in a loss of 100 pounds in a year. Much to her surprise, she had come to view herself as a person who exercises. She communicated this belief to her children sufficiently that when a teacher gave a sentence completion to the classroom, her son responded: "My mother . . . exercises."
>
> Alice also lost enough weight that she once again began encountering the issues that had precipitated her weight gain in the first place—issues of low self-worth and sexuality. She was at considerable risk for relapse unless these psychological issues were addressed directly.
>
> A combination of life changes, therapy changes, increases in anxiety and depression, and the failure of medication to control these symptoms, precipitated a decrease in exercise and some weight regain. The key relapse questions, mentioned above, were crucial in assisting Alice to learn from her recent experience rather than return to her prior sense of herself as a failure.

The theoretical framework described here becomes, in the next chapter, a basis for the pragmatics of developing exercise plans with clients. It is assumed that the vast majority of psychotherapy clients do not currently exercise and thus that most are precontemplators, contemplators, or, perhaps, preparers.

The Pragmatics of Exercise Initiation and Maintenance | 5

E xercise can be a challenging undertaking. In contrast to medication, a passive therapy with low demand on the client and an external agent as the active ingredient, exercise is an active therapy that makes high demands on the client, the agent of the effect. "To follow the exercise prescription, the client must (a) overcome inertia to start motion; (b) make a choice of activity including location, time, etc.; and (c) continue what some describe to be the effortful, sometimes painful process of movement" (Sime, 1996, p. 163). Engaging the client in this process, then, also can be a challenge.

Clients enter therapy at various stages of exercise involvement. In this chapter I focus primarily on issues relevant to clients who are not currently exercising, although concerns about exercise maintenance and the management of relapse need to be taken into consideration at all stages of exercise engagement. Through the synergistic blending of general knowledge about exercise efficacy and the particulars of a person's life, the creativity of therapy allows for an individually tailored exercise prescription.

In this process, it is critical to retain one's role as a psychotherapist, not as a physician or a coach. The therapist should ensure that clients have taken appropriate steps, such as visiting their physician, to evaluate their own physical capacity to embark on any increase in physical activity. Likewise, if the form of exercise chosen involves specific training or unfamiliar equipment, clients should be referred to a personal trainer, instructor, or coach.

Throughout the process of exercise initiation and continuation, it is vital to help clients attend to the ways in which they are mentally monitoring their exercise behaviors. It is helpful to review with clients what they are saying to themselves about themselves, and the degree to which these internal assumptions or dialogues serve to enhance self-esteem and self-efficacy as well as bolster exercise habits. As with any other aspect of behavior—especially in its initial stages—considerable information can be gleaned and, if necessary, course correction can be implemented.

> 32-year-old Glenna had been sinking into a continuously deeper and increasingly enervating depression over a period of weeks. As her emotional life unraveled, she found it difficult to get to (professional) work in the morning. Making meals was effortful; washing and combing her long and attractive hair became more than she could tolerate. As the weekend approached, with forecasts of weather conditions ideal for skiing, we discussed ways she could cope with the weekend. An expert skier, Glenna planned a day on the slopes.
>
> When she returned early the following week, Glenna's mood, energy, and self-esteem were no higher than before. When asked, she reported that she had spent hours cross-country skiing—and had accompanied the rhythm of the glide with the chant *"sickie, sickie, sickie."* A potentially pleasurable and energizing time had instead been held hostage to and incorporated into her pervasive negative self-evaluation. Clearly, exercise at this time was insufficient to counter her depression.

In the sections that follow, I make specific suggestions with regard to the most salient parameters in exercise initiation and maintenance, and the management of relapse. These suggestions are drawn from the theoretical and research literatures as well as clinical practice. Appendix C, The Exercise History and Motivation Inventory and Exercise Plan, reflects these points and can be used directly with clients.

Helping Clients Get Started

The best place to begin discussion of exercise is often during the intake interview (Sime, 1996). As the therapist does with other questions related to the client's current functioning, she or he can ask about both current and past type and level of physical activity, as well as interest in and enjoyment from these activities. These general questions give the therapist a sense of the stage of change the client is in, self-efficacy for exercise, readiness to develop new exercise behaviors, and initial barriers to change.

In suggesting exercise to clients for the first time, Johnsgard (1989) emphasizes four points to clients: exercise will help; exercise reduces depression quickly; moderation and flexibility are critical; and patients have the resources to independently find relief from their symptoms. Clients are thus given both information and a sense of hope, each critical to the therapy process.

TYPE OF EXERCISE

Berger (1994) developed an initial exercise taxonomy, designed to highlight those aspects of exercise that are most conducive to mood-enhancing effects. To the extent that these are maximized, they may serve as internal reinforcers that will assist in the initiation and maintenance of exercise. The three major requirements are (a) that the activity be pleasing and enjoyable; (b) that the mode be aerobic or involve rhythmical abdominal breathing, and that the activity be predictable or spatially certain, with an absence of interpersonal competition; and (c) that the exercise be regularly included in one's weekly schedule, of moderate intensity, and of at least 20 to 30 minutes duration.

Although much of the research on exercise and mood has been in relation to running, other forms of exercise, including swimming and hatha yoga, meet the taxonomy criteria as well (Berger & Owen, 1986, 1992a). Activities that are repetitive and do not require much attention in and of themselves allow one to tune out and tune in. However, to some degree this is a function of people's capacity to tolerate the boredom and routine of these forms of exercise. People who regularly perform aerobic forms of exercise will often find diversity in minutiae and describe the predictability as allowing for variety. The most effective exercise will be that which takes into account individual characteristics and matches these characteristics to the exercise prescription. "Exercise can be solitary, social, competitive, or easygoing. . . . Treatment variety is a significant strength of exercise therapy" (Johnsgard, 1989, p. 149). An attitude of curiosity on the part of the client and "collaborative empiricism" (Beck, Rush, Hollon, & Shaw, 1979) on the part of the therapist allows this matching process to be one of discovery.

> I usually encourage exercise, but I tend to be cautious in the way that I push it. Different people have different ways of achieving the goals I achieve through exercise. Many times the suggestion to exercise is experienced as another should. I don't find shoulds helpful. The kind of benefits I receive come from discovering how exercise works for me individually, and likewise benefits are individualized for others.
>
> **34-year-old female clinical social worker**

DOSE OR FIT OF EXERCISE

The cardiovascular prescription of exercise three to five times per week, of moderate intensity, lasting 20–40 minutes, often has been transferred to an appropriate mental dose as well. The exercise parameters of frequency (F), intensity (I), and duration or time (T) can be remembered as the acronym FIT.

FIT also refers to the process of exercise initiation and change. The general principle is to vary only one of these dimensions at a time. Although some practitioners (Kirschenbaum, 1994; Lesyk, 1998) recommend daily exercise (starting at low intensity or duration), I tend to recommend some initial flexibility regarding frequency. Shifting from exercising no days a week to 7 days can be a large leap. The expectation that one must exercise 7 days days a week can result in discontinuing if one misses a day. For people who have not routinely exercised, a day without exercise may be immediately interpreted as "Aha! I knew it. A failure again. I can't stick with anything." Anticipating the need for a certain amount of slack helps clients appreciate their humanness. On the other hand, exercising less frequently than three times a week can lead to too many rationalizations, the lack of development of habit, inefficiency, and muscle soreness with each exercise episode. A decrease in chronic mental benefits also may be experienced.

Perceived effort, which appears related to self-efficacy for exercise, may be an effective means of monitoring exercise intensity (Rudolph & McAuley, 1996). One can measure perceived exertion using Borg's Ratings of Perceived Exertion (RPE) scale (Borg, 1985), with a range from 6 to 20 that reflects self-perception of exertion and fatigue. Informally, a client may be encouraged to measure his or her mental effort and fatigue on a 10-point scale. A person initiating a program of exercise will experience it as effortful. In general, from a training perspective, initial intensity should start fairly low. By focusing on perceived effort, or preferred effort (Dishman, 1994b), the client can begin assessing the level of intensity that appears to have the most positive mood effect.

Another easily adaptable method of determining the intensity of effort is the talk test, the ability to maintain a conversation (if desired) while exercising (Berger, 1984b; Sime & Sanstead, 1987). If it takes longer than an hour to recover from a single session of exercise, either the intensity or the duration should be decreased.

Although some studies have found a dose-response interaction (that is, the more intense, the greater the response), a number of other studies have not found such a relationship (Sime, 1996). After a certain amount of training, clients may habituate to a particular level of exercise intensity. If that occurs, they may find that they again experience the physiological kick or psychological response, or both, if they vary the intensity. The increased exertion may augment the distraction afforded by activity.

The duration, or length of time, that one exercises, tends to be one of the variables most noticeable to a client, and therefore potentially of value in changes of self-perception. Incremental increases in stamina are quantifiable, and thus are indicators of the changes the client has made. However, a client who thinks: "I should be able to run for a half hour without feeling winded, since I've been exercising for three weeks now" will receive few psychological benefits because his or her expectation is unrealistic. One of the most frequent reasons that people stop exercising is because of changes in the FIT that are too rapid—especially a too rapid increase in duration. Standard advice to runners is to increase any variable no more than 10% per week. This percentage change seems agonizingly slow to many people, yet it increases the likelihood that the client will be injury free, allows for physiological adaptation, and supports the positive effect of persistence. The therapist can reassure the client that shorter periods of exercise also are efficacious. For example, even 15 minutes of vigorous aerobic exercise can result in significant anxiety reduction (Petruzello & Landers, 1994).

FIT is also a concept that can be used metaphorically to describe movement in the change process. Thus, a person in preparation may recognize FIT through more frequent thoughts of the benefits of exercise, or recollection of a particularly pleasurable past exercise experience, or the actual experience of exercising for a bit longer. Likewise, in assessing depression, a person may notice that in the past month they sighed less frequently, or did not feel as down, or that their level of energy lasted longer.

EXERCISE HISTORY, VALUES, AND BELIEFS

Understanding clients' exercise history as well as exploring their beliefs about themselves and exercise are critical issues when working with them to develop patterns of exercise with which they are likely to become involved. What type of exercise have they enjoyed in the past? What have they wanted to do but haven't tried? What kind of activity has meaning to them (Wankel, 1993)? What types of exercise take salient personal variables into account (e.g., risk-taking or predictability, sociability and need or desire to be socially engaged, financial flexibility)? How likely do they think it is that they will actually begin and continue exercising at this time (self-efficacy)?

Although a history of activity tends to predict the likelihood of future activity, it also is important to recognize that such history may have been reified or romanticized. For example, a therapist may want to attend to ways in which a former jock competes internally against his image of who he was 20 years ago. Inevitably (out of shape and older), he will lose if this is his initial standard today.

MATCHING THE EXERCISE PLAN TO THE PROBLEM

Johnsgard (1989) suggested that one of the important determinants of exercise should be the type of problem for which the client is seeking help. Thus, the high stress client may find it most useful to develop a program that will reduce resting heart rate and blood pressure and to plan activity during a midday break in the midst of a stressful work day. Alternatively, the client can learn to use the same form of exercise for different purposes:

> Alice, described more fully in chapter 6, began using a stationary bicycle as part of the treatment plan for management of depression, anxiety, and posttraumatic stress disorder. Daily low level cycling for 20 minutes had little effect. She increased the frequency to three times a day (and thus, the duration as well), and varied the intensity. In the morning, she would ride the bicycle for 15 minutes to become more alert and control panic. She used this time, also, to visualize methods for coping with the day. In the afternoon, she pedaled at high intensity for 15 minutes, to alleviate the stresses of work and as an alternative to binge eating. In the evening, slow and comfortable, she rode for varying lengths of time as she reworked trauma issues.

SOCIOCULTURAL VARIABLES

Gender differences in how men and women are socialized with regard to exercise, as well as current cultural expectations, are especially significant as clients consider exercise. Some women are initially uncomfortable with the (new) experience of salty sweat in their eyes. Some men appear constitutionally incapable of running without timing themselves, measuring themselves against an internal standard, and continually trying for a personal best.

In a community sample, prediction of exercise adoption over a 2-year period varied by sex. Among sedentary men, exercise adoption related to self-efficacy, age (negative), and neighborhood environment. Women's exercise adoption was predicted by level of education, self-efficacy, and friend and family support for exercise (Sallis et al., 1992).

Exercise has been popularized as a middle-class, White activity. Unfortunately, not much information is available concerning exercise in relation to class or ethnicity (Dishman, 1994a; Hall, 1998).

SOCIAL SUPPORTS

This is a complex and somewhat idiosyncratic variable: The right social supports are wonderful; the wrong ones, devastating. Social supports may include one's family members, friends, colleagues, or exercise buddies.

> The advantages of recommending exercise to clients include:
>
> 1. Immediate sense of increased physical efficacy;
> 2. Perception of greater involvement in their life;
> 3. Doing something selfish that is good for you and can serve as a bridge to an improved sense of self-worth;
> 4. Establishing and developing a new interest serves to distract from problems (which are always gonna be there);
> 5. Likely to meet new acquaintances.
>
> **50-year-old male psychologist**

Particularly in the middle stages of change (contemplation and preparation), the warmth and empathy of others are critically important (Prochaska, Norcross, & DiClemente, 1994). And many programs emphasize the importance of social interaction in developing exercise habits (Dishman, 1994a). "Individuals are attracted to group activity for a number of reasons, including: group identification and commitment, social reinforcement, competitive stimulation and the opportunity for team activities" (Wan-kel, 1993, p. 155). Regular contact with members of an exercise class, or locker room connections, or genuine family support, can all bolster one's self-esteem or sustain flagging energy. But negative reactions or invidious comparison can deter or dampen one's enthusiasm. This, then, is an area in which to listen carefully and be especially attuned to clients' particular thoughts, feelings, and experiences.

Some people look to exercise as a time for relationship. For others, exercise may be a socially sanctioned opportunity for disconnection. Women overburdened with child-care responsibilities or the social commerce of life, for example, may experience legitimate solitude as a sought-after luxury. That this desire is not entirely gendered is illustrated by New York City Ballet dancer Edward Liang, who commented, "It's . . . soothing to work out because it's for you. It's time to be by yourself. It's my time away from everybody else" (Martins & Kaplan, 1997).

ENVIRONMENTAL FACTORS

Whether perceived or actual, environmental barriers are among the most significant deterrents to exercise adoption and continuance. These may involve issues of access, such as physical location or expense (Dishman, 1994a), or the logistics of squeezing yet one more thing into an already full day. Alternatively, the therapist and client can reassess the obligatory implications of exercise. Increased physical activity, incorporated into daily living, can assist the client in feeling more efficient and decrease the experience of exercise as a demand on one's all too precious available time (Sime, 1996).

> Usually I do solo workouts, as I schedule them during my work day. Working out is my time out from others and responsibilities. The silence is golden.
>
> **44-year-old female psychologist**

Although there are standard (and often legitimate) barriers to exercise, there are also individual differences concerning those barriers. In a study of three different population types, Godin et al. (1994) noted differences in perceived barriers to exercise, even among those with a high intention to exercise. Among members of the general population, perceived difficulty to find time was the strongest barrier. People with coronary heart disease (CHD) were concerned about lack of access to a specialized exercise center, restrictions by their physician, or heart pain. Pregnant women anticipated concern about their baby's physical health and problems with time management.

It is often with the minutiae that a therapist can be most creative in helping a client identify and overcome potential barriers. Although there appears to be no specific psychobiological best time of day to exercise (O'Connor & Davis, 1992), discussion with a client regarding when or where to exercise, for example, can be very productive.

Gordon, described more fully in chapter 8, developed a regular routine of going to the gym to exercise on his way home from work. Yet, insecure about his work performance, he tended to arrive at work on Mondays, the first day of the work week, highly anxious. Exercising before work on Mondays alleviated much of his tension.

Exercise Adherence

The term *compliance* suggests that a participant is following recommendations or prescription from an authority figure. An expectation of compliance may evoke a variety of issues around noncompliance, including control by another, passivity, and external locus of control. In contrast, it has been suggested that the terms *adherence* and *nonadherence* describe free choice, in which the person is participating, acting, and able to maintain an internal locus of control (Meichenbaum & Turk, 1987).

Some people find just the right exercise and have no trouble with exercise adherence. Whether they have been able to guess right, or learn from past experience, or serendipity happens, they experience a match between person and exercise. When that occurs, the issue of motivation becomes moot, for the exercise itself provides all the reinforcement that is needed. The interaction of challenge, expectation, clear feedback, focused attention, and absorption in the activity results in a sense of deep pleasure. Enjoyment (i.e., intrinsic motivation) is a central variable that affects exercise adherence and improved psychological well-being (Wankel, 1993).

Since not everyone experiences enjoyment at all, or the first time, exercise adherence can often be an issue. Predictably, 50% of people stop exercising within 6 months of beginning an exercise program (Dishman, 1988). As mentioned, this dropout pattern is similar to adherence rates for any health behavior change (Meichenbaum & Turk, 1987). Although not a cause for alarm, it is worth a great deal of attention, however, especially when developing individualized plans with clients. How, then, can a therapist help clients continue or renew their exercising?

An attitude of curiosity or experimentation is vital in beginning and continuing the exercise adventure. This approach serves in and of itself to counteract the hopelessness of depression or the tension of anxiety. Further, it allows a client to attend dispassionately to the effects of exercise and internalize those effects.

Once clients are exercising regularly, it is important to help them develop a system to monitor the exercise. Keeping a record, whether in a diary or on a chart, complex or simple, serves numerous functions (Berger, 1984b). It is both a reinforcer and a basis for information. A log can serve as a source of motivation, a method of immediate and positive reinforcement, a chronicle of progress, a location for problem description and resolution, and an indication of program adherence (thus subject to positive reinforcement from others). Since human memory is both objectively and subjectively fallible, a written record serves as a sentinel of reality. The client who disparages having walked for only 15 minutes can be referred back to her own record: 2 weeks ago, she felt winded after walking for 10 minutes. Exercise monitoring also can allow the person to assess and reassess current functioning and make changes in type of exercise as appropriate.

Although goal setting can be useful in exercise initiation, this process may be vital to exercise maintenance. Standard recommendations for setting goals that are realistic, behaviorally specific, and over which one has control apply with regard to exercise initiation and maintenance. In addition, setting multiple goals means that the client does not stand or fall on the basis of only one parameter. Goals that describe an acceptable range may provide a supportive combination of specificity and flexibility. For example, a client may set goals relating to minimal or maximal hours of exercise per week, or a range of miles walked per week. The process of developing that range can be interesting in and of itself, and involve the client in direct observation of his or her own body's capacity. Both short- and long-term goals are important. Short-term goals provide immediate reinforcement, whereas long-term goals support sustainable perspective. Clients may find it helpful to remember the acronym SMART, for goals that are Specific, Measurable, Action-oriented, Realistic, and Timed.

The goal setting described thus far refers to the what of exercise. Goals also reflect the why of exercise. Although health-related goals often are reported as most important, they have not been found to distinguish between adherers and dropouts of exercise. On the other hand, non-health related goals, such as developing recreational skills, social relationships, and satisfying one's curiosity, have been found to differentiate adherers from dropouts (Wankel, 1993).

Motivation for exercise often changes over time. Take, for example, running. Reporting both on a study of members of the Fifty-Plus Runners' Association and a *Running Times* magazine survey, Johnsgard commented that although there are some gender differences in motive,

> being lean and fit become taken for granted—accomplishments which will persist as a part of a new lifestyle. . . . As . . . [the] weeks roll by, psychological benefits are realized and become central motives. These increasingly strong motives have to do with how we feel about ourselves and with how we feel, our emotional moods. They become basic in sustaining regular training for both sexes. (1989, p. 49)

As people become more aware of the variety of psychological benefits of exercise, they become able to use exercise to suit their purpose:

> When 38-year-old Rebecca began running for weight management, she did not anticipate the stress-reducing effects that she found herself experiencing. In her journal, she began sketching longer and longer lines (indicating running) and shorter and shorter dashes (describing walking) to illustrate her increasing running duration. Often, she would add notes about thoughts and images she had had while running. She wrote down her body measurements, and noticed changes in body

shape even more than weight. Committed to running, when she experienced some major life stressors she deliberately paid attention to the ways in which running alleviated her stress.

Relapse

Relapse may not be entirely preventable, but the degree of backsliding can be addressed. Much of this has to do with what one says to oneself about oneself, what one believes about oneself.

One of the best methods of relapse prevention is relapse prediction. A therapist may comment to a client, "Many people stop and resume exercising a number of times before developing a regular pattern of exercise. What situations may get you off track? How long would it last? What would help get you started again?" These questions allow clients to think ahead, to take responsibility for their exercising, and to understand some of the motivational forces that are central to their exercising. Most typically, these issues involve pattern shifts: weather, other participants' changes in routine, illness or injury, vacation, and so forth. The other major predictor of relapse is sameness (i.e., boredom). A sense of stagnation can be understood as an opportunity to assess clients' reasons for exercising, reasons that may differ from those for initiating exercise. A client may find it useful to develop a new decisional balance scale. Clients also can use their observing self to discover new angles to old behavior, mindfulness, for example, rather than mindlessness.

> At intake, 45-year-old Connie reported a period of a few months during which she had bicycled regularly and enjoyed it immensely. A leg injury brought the biking to a halt. She was feeling extremely discouraged by a ride a few days previously, during which she found she could only ride a block before she became winded and her legs began aching. She seemed to be waiting until, in some magical way, she would be transported back to the pre-injury time. Instead, I encouraged her to resume riding at the level at which her body was currently functioning, and increase the distance only very gradually.

There also may be times when it is useful to help clients start with a clean slate, reassessing their priorities entirely. Erickson's principle of resistance utilization (Erickson, Rossi, & Rossi, 1976), the Eastern martial arts, or Merle Jordan's (1986) concept of "going in the direction that the camel is already headed," each allow relapse to become an opportunity for new understanding and change.

Janice, a 37-year-old professional with three young children, sought therapy because she was feeling overwhelmed and recognized that she was not taking care of herself adequately. There were days when she wouldn't brush her teeth, shower, or exercise, despite knowing that she liked the way that it felt to take care of herself. "I sabotage myself," she admitted. Compounding the situation, she found herself lying to her husband, an avid exerciser, telling him she had exercised when she hadn't. The more she described her life stresses, the demands she placed on herself, and her distress and guilt, the more it suggested to me reversing my more typical recommendation. I encouraged her to give herself time off from exercise expectation. Her immediate response was a feeling of great relief.

At the next session, we discussed how to contain this time off. Janice had described an all-or-nothing style in which she would make a strong commitment and then drop out of activities, giving up on herself. This time, I suggested that she set a date by which she would review her decision. In this way, she would not feel a free-floating anxiety that would then result in new guilt and paralysis. Immediately, she picked a date 3 weeks hence. She also decided to claim a personal "retreat" day to reflect: during half of the day she would review her personal life plans, and during the other half, the work decisions she needed to make.

During that "retreat" week, she came in for a session and reported that she had specifically not exercised for 2 weeks. She now was starting to rebuild from the ground up. She and her husband were incorporating a regular weekly ski time together. She could reestablish an enjoyable tennis time with a friend. And then she could just decide to do some form of exercise on the weekends. Her husband, she recognized, used some of his weekend time in this way, and would certainly support her in such a plan.

In the next chapter, the focus shifts to the use of exercise during the psychotherapy hour itself. The change in the location of treatment may have applicability for clients at any level of commitment to exercise.

Walking the Walk While Talking the Talk:
Exercising With Clients

6

T he concept of conducting psychotherapy during times of physical activity dates back at least to Anna Freud's development of play therapy (1928). Using physical activity as the therapeutic method or as a means to therapeutic connection is a traditional form of treatment for children and adolescents. Yet physical activity with adults, when it occurs at all in conjunction with mental health, is generally consigned to recreation therapy within institutions. For the most part, neither the burgeoning field of applied sport psychology nor more traditional psychotherapies have further developed the reciprocally beneficial possibilities of this particular mix.

Because of this paucity of information, and because of the synergistic potential of exercise during psychotherapy, in this chapter I provide a framework for considering exercising with clients during therapy and present some detailed case descriptions.

Exercise in Psychotherapy

Exercise incorporated into psychotherapy may be considered a tool of therapy in the same manner as free association or desensitization (Barnes, 1980). "If we think of psychotherapy as being like gardening, then the psychotherapist is the gardener. And gardeners use many tools:

mechanical, chemical, heuristic, and at times spiritual. Running is a new psychotherapeutic tool that may change both the garden and the gardener" (Kostrubala,1984, p. 124). Popularized by Kostrubala (1977), the combination of exercise and verbal therapy, conducted simultaneously, received a flurry of anecdotal attention in the early 1980s (Sachs & Buffone, 1984; Sacks & Sachs, 1981), but experimental research has been lacking (Johnsgard, 1989).

Although the beneficial effects of a number of kinds of exercise have been examined, for both historical and practical reasons, running has been the form of exercise most frequently described in relation to exercise and mental health (Sachs, 1984b; Sime & Sanstead, 1987). Perhaps as a consequence, the terms *exercise therapy* and *running therapy* have been used at times interchangeably, adding semantic confusion to a field already lacking experimental precision. Further, exercise therapy at times describes exercise alone, yet with an adjectival implication of the impact of exercise on the psyche. Because of these various confusions in terminology, I refer in this chapter to both exercise and therapy when the two are used together.

Walking or jogging are generally the preferred forms of exercise during the therapy session. The setting is readily available, this type of exercise requires no special equipment beyond appropriate footwear, and little training is needed. Most significant, client and therapist can exercise and talk simultaneously. (Clearly, if therapy is going to occur while running, both client and therapist will need to be sufficiently fit to both run and talk.)

The psychological value of exercise in psychotherapy is apparent. "Even brisk walking on the part of unconditioned patients seems to 'loosen them up.' They become less inhibited and constrained and more in touch with their immediate feelings and experience" (Johnsgard, 1989, p. 169). Johnsgard further observed that his patients had more energy, were more aware of anger and assertive needs, talked about what they genuinely felt (in contrast to what they thought they should feel), and were more conscious of themselves yet less self-inhibited or self-conscious.

Exercising with clients has the additional advantage of potentially supporting client initiation and maintenance of exercise itself (Johnsgard, 1989; Sime, 1996), with its attendant physiological and psychological benefits.

Lacking theory or empirical investigation regarding the use of exercise in psychotherapy, yet considering the potential salubrious effects, there may be some common characteristics and issues that inhere to this form of psychotherapy. It is important to recognize that the more active the movement, the further this form of treatment shifts from the typical bounds and constraints of psychotherapy. In the commentary that follows, then, it is suggested that running with clients, for example, poses potentially more risk along the various dimensions described than does walking with clients. Since there is so little experimental research on the subject, it is not clear whether the benefits to exercising with clients, let alone running with them, outweigh these risks. Johnsgard (1989), however, has suggested that increased access to deep affect may be part of the power of running during therapy.

There are at present no guidelines for therapists with regard to exercise during therapy. Certain demand characteristics (i.e., creativity, energy, physical conditioning, and a style of openness to interpersonal, interactive, and participative therapy) seem apparent. Since this is an elaboration and extension of psychotherapy, the therapist must first be thoroughly skilled in conducting psychotherapy. There is no information to suggest that a particular therapeutic orientation would be more or less beneficial. Running has been used in combination with psychoanalysis, cognitive-behavior therapy, hypnosis, guided imagery, and generic counseling (Buffone, 1984b). Knowledge of applied sport science, although potentially useful, does not appear critically necessary.

> Exercise is a natural way to build social support. I think clients can really feel good when they take on a new activity and potentially make new exercise partners. Exercising with clients during therapy could promote dependency. Therapists should believe in a client's ability to engage in activity when s/he is ready. I often have impulses to want to help clients by exercising with them, but I think the underlying message would be that they don't have the capacity to achieve this on their own.
>
> **30-year-old female psychologist**

Any therapy on the borders of the known and approved obligates the practitioner to be fully conscious of the limits of one's skills and competence, and to be especially mindful concerning ethical principles and guidelines (APA, 1992). Certain general principles of ethics have specific application in the sport and exercise context (Sachs, 1993). In this type of therapy, it may be particularly important to have peer if not formal supervision, so that the therapist can assess various real and potential issues in a reflective environment.

A therapist who was an avid horseback rider and owned two horses considered suggesting a riding-therapy session to one of her clients. This client had a love of riding but had been financially constrained from riding for the past few years. The therapist thought that this experience might provide an element missing from the client's life and be a setting conducive to therapeutic work. Additionally, her horses would get a workout that they needed.

Hesitant about using this new therapeutic modality, however, the therapist consulted with a peer supervision group.

Her colleagues, including me (even though I am an advocate of the judicious combination of exercise with psychotherapy), were all markedly concerned. Although the therapist's motives were altruistic, she was potentially increasing the client's dependence on her, was markedly changing the therapeutic boundary by having the client come to her home, and was dramatically increasing her liability risk of injury to the client. Her colleagues endorsed her alternative idea: to support ways in which her client might find a stable where she could ride in exchange for cleaning stalls and grooming horses.

In the sections that follow, certain aspects of exercise during therapy are highlighted, along with interpersonal issues that need to be kept in the therapist's consciousness. I have described some of these issues and features in more detail elsewhere (Hays, 1994b). Specific case examples of walking and running during therapy are then described.

Special Characteristics of Exercise During Therapy

Among qualities of activity that may heighten the therapeutic experience are changes in thinking patterns, the use of symbolism and metaphor, and nonverbal communication.

Clarity of thinking and capacity to synthesize in new ways is a phenomenon that may be particularly accessible to a person either while active or within a short time afterward. Rarely described, defined, or commented on, and notoriously challenging to researchers (Sachs, 1984a), this shift in thinking is an experience known to many runners. For a number of people, this cognitive component is an integral aspect to exercise maintenance. It is as if one has increased access to mental processes. The kinds of thinking typically associated with the right brain—integrative, intuitive, holistic—seem more available to processing by the left brain. For lack of a better term, one may refer to this synthesis as right-brain problem solving. The ways in which this increased productivity and creativity may enhance the therapeutic process have been only occasionally explored (Murphy, 1996).

The prophylactic and mood-elevating effects of exercise, as well as an increased capacity for lucidity of thought and potential for cognitive integration, may be accessible to the therapist as well as client. The cognitive shifts that occur for the therapist have implications beyond the immediate client session. To the extent that the centering effect lasts for some time after the actual exercising, the next client or clients also may benefit. With a heightened sense of well-being, the therapist may feel less overwhelmed by later patients' symptoms (e.g., the contagion of depression), as well as more energetic, relaxed, and focused (Buffone, 1984c; Johnsgard, 1989).

> On long runs I seem to be able to pull together information in novel ways, by letting go of consciously linear thinking patterns. On the surface, these may appear as random thoughts, yet they end up coming together in delightful and meaningful ways. For example, I come up with some of my best paper and presentation titles while running. The problem is, of course, in order to use any of these great ideas you have to remember them long enough to get through the rest of the run and get back to a pen and paper.
>
> The extraordinary part of this is that it is so effortless and perhaps that it happens at all. The kind of thinking that we spend years developing in graduate school is so taxing, time consuming, linear. Perhaps Jung was correct after all. Rational, linear, conscious thinking takes effort and is not the way the brain naturally processes information. It is this dreamlike thinking—for lack of a better descriptor—that is the way we usually process information. We've just learned to ignore and devalue it.
>
> **40-year-old male psychologist**

Because the mode of expression is physical, exercise therapy contains many opportunities for symbolic and metaphoric representation of issues, conflicts, and resolutions (Gleser & Brown, 1988; Gologor, 1979). Since one of the most effective means of communicating with clients is to use language that has salience to them and their experience, exercise language as metaphor is particularly rich in possibility—whether or not one is actually exercising with the client. One can talk about pacing oneself, or developing a rhythm. Symbolic or metaphoric descriptions of exercise can, additionally, assist the resolution of resistance or defensiveness (Hays, 1993).

Just as the therapist attends to nonverbal forms of communication in office therapy, the movement of exercise offers an excellent opportunity to gain and use information from a variety of unspoken sources. Because the language of exercise is the body, body awareness serves several functions. Body signals can cue clients to information below consciousness; the value of attention to the present moment is underscored; the activity encourages an integration of mind and body. For survivors of bodily assault, integration of mind and body can be especially healing (Herman, 1992).

Therapists should be attuned to the potential that increased activity and body awareness could be the locus for flashbacks or body memories (Freyd, 1996). There is no reported information that this has occurred, nor have I experienced it in the trauma work that I have done. If it were to arise, the skilled trauma therapist could use such an experience as an opportunity for further trauma resolution.

Reflecting on the mind-body connection, Polly, a client described more fully below, noted:

> Running during therapy feels like a very active form of learning. I process information through my body and from there to my mind, and then it gets integrated. The physical sensations are like a feedback loop which serves to validate and confirm my feelings. Sometimes part of the run is very difficult—the idea/issue we discuss may be difficult for me to grasp or upset me emotionally. When that happens my breathing and pulse increase, my stride shortens—all the symptoms of being physically stressed. During my athletic training I've learned to "listen" to the physical signs and respond accordingly—I try to slow the rate of my breathing, lengthen my stride, and run from a centered point in my body. My physical "observer" has been active for a long time—now I'm learning to listen to my emotions. I'm really at a point where awareness is important and being aware of my body has helped me be aware of my feelings. (Hays, 1994b, p. 732)

Interpersonal Issues in Exercise During Therapy

Exercising during therapy heightens certain therapeutic issues and potentially alters the therapeutic contract. This therapy differs dramatically from traditional psychotherapy through shared activity, resulting in a more equal balance between therapist and client. It is therefore especially important to attend to client and therapist characteristics and changes in the interpersonal frame. Although some of the interpersonal issues described below refer to the client rather than the therapist, the therapist always retains responsibility for creating and maintaining boundaries so that a harmful dual role relationship does not develop.

Part of the appeal—and therefore part of the hazard—of exercising in therapy is that by its nature the interaction between therapist and client is changed. It is useful, then, to spell out a number of implications and cautions. Given these constraints, this type of therapy may have a narrower range of utility than initially thought. It appears that optimal use of this type of therapy involves thoughtful attention to the combination of client and therapist characteristics as well as adaptations to the therapeutic frame.

Logistically, there are basic issues of organization and physiology. Are changes of clothing required, and how are those handled? Are both client and therapist sufficiently fit to carry on conversation while moving? Can they accommodate one another's pace and converse at the same time? The greater the level of activity, the more relevant these questions become.

From a psychological perspective, how are diagnostic and interpersonal issues addressed? Without guidelines, training, or protocols, how does the therapist assess the appropriate client intervention? How do client and therapist handle boundaries, intimacy, competition, eroticization, and power? How does the increased openness and parity of shared activity fit the therapist's style? Where are limits set? How are potential ethical concerns and the possibility of exploitation handled? Most centrally, do the purported benefits of this therapy suit the client's needs?

> One hazard of exercising with clients is the potential for ambiguity or the development of relationship problems with the client. This may be "dual relationship" stuff, or perhaps sexual arousal (or either or both). With a mature, focused therapist who is aware of boundaries and capable of enforcing them, this risk can be minimized.
>
> **55-year-old male psychologist**

These questions do not have definitive or absolute answers. It behooves the therapist to anticipate potential issues and have sufficient collegial support to maintain ongoing self-reflection.

CLIENT ISSUES

A number of issues are particularly relevant to the client. Is the client able to use exercise as the medium in which psychotherapy occurs, rather than the focus of the therapy? This may be a function of both the client's fitness and the role of activity in the client's life. When working with an already committed exerciser, some of the potentially complicating factors around training, coaching, and adherence, all of which offer a variety of pitfalls and mixed role relationships, may be obviated.

To what degree does physical activity allow the client to avoid the emotion rather than confront it and work it through? In therapy, there is a continuous tension between containment and expression. Theoretical and stylistic differences in approach, as well as specific therapist-client interactions, help define the optimal balance (Hollander-Goldfein, Fosshage, & Bahr, 1989). As illustrated in the case descriptions below and elsewhere (Hays, 1994b; Hays, 1996), my own experience suggests that the medium of physical activity can allow the expression and resolution of affects otherwise blocked.

The therapist, nonetheless, should be alert to the potential that exercise during therapy may be used for pathological purposes. Those at particular risk may be clients presenting with problems of eating disorders, obsessive-compulsive characteristics, or those who already overuse exercise (Thompson, 1993; Yates, 1991).

THERAPIST ISSUES

Certain therapist issues are especially salient as well. Relying on sessions for one's own exercise both heightens the value of the session beyond its intrinsic value and may result in inappropriate and disproportionate disappointment if plans change. There is no reason to believe that therapists who exercise are any different from the general public in their potential to overuse exercise (Raglin, 1990). The therapist exercising with a client thus needs to retain a balanced perspective on exercise and to have alternatives available.

In our litigious society, with an ever-expanding variety of therapeutic techniques of dubious value, additional issues should be assessed. Are there liability issues specific to this form of therapy? Are there potential breaches of confidentiality if the therapist works with the client outside of the office? The responsible therapist assesses these issues in the context of the specific case, seeking consultation where appropriate, and reviewing issues as necessary with the client.

In sharing an activity with the client, the therapist becomes more known as a person. The reality of the therapist is more evident; body, pacing, self-pacing, and windedness are some obvious examples. Additionally, the atmosphere of shared activity may in and of itself evoke increased self-disclosure by the therapist (Kostrubala, 1977). Although not necessarily inappropriate, the therapist needs to recognize these effects and monitor them continually. Depending on therapist and type of therapy, the increased visibility of the therapist's self may be more or less comfortable. Regardless, as with therapist disclosure in an office setting, the client's benefit must be the object (Kroll, 1988).

> This is a very tricky area, primarily because it is outside of the conventional boundaries of therapy. I feel this should only be done if a therapist is clear about what he or she is doing and clear about their personal gratification in doing this. I think the therapist should have a clear therapeutic rationale for it and should be able to articulate that to the client (and the licensing board if need be).
>
> One cannot always predict (or even understand in retrospect) how a client interprets boundary crossings, even if the therapist is totally clear about such things.
>
> I think exercising with a client probably would be inadvisable in any cases in which there is a strong attraction or attachment on the part of the client.
>
> **51-year-old female psychologist**

INTERPERSONAL ISSUES

When engaging in activity as part of psychotherapy, the therapist needs to attend to a number of interpersonal issues. As with any interpersonal engagement, the therapist should be aware of issues regarding power, competition, and sexuality. By encouraging or supporting exercise during therapy, the therapist is exerting power and influence. Attempting to please the therapist, the client may accede to exercise during therapy.

> A year after individual therapy with 41-year-old Lenore was completed, I heard some disquieting information from her group therapist. Lenore had recently disclosed that she had felt obligated to walk during therapy in order to please me. This information ran counter to my perception of our work together: Lenore had appeared interested in walking during therapy and had been the one who suggested that it become our normal routine. The combination of walking and talking had seemed synergistic. Yet perhaps Lenore's current description reflected a level of anger and passive aggressiveness that was never touched in individual therapy. Or possibly she was playing bad therapist-good therapist. Regardless, this information reminded me of the complexity of the therapeutic endeavor, with all its layers of meaning.

The potential for competition between therapist and client also should be recognized. The specific gender pairing is especially relevant in this regard. Although women are socialized in our culture to be less overtly competitive than men, in the context of therapy more subtle forms of competition may be all the more salient. Socialization to sport competition is in itself a particular subset of competition and has its own rules, specific to gender and culture (Gill, 1993). The cultural isomorphism between sport, competition, and masculinity (Oglesby & Hill, 1993) suggests the following possible interpersonal dynamics with running therapy. Physically active men may be more likely to be ego-involved in the activity, and thus the potential for competition will be strong. Altshul (1981), a psychiatrist, provided a poignant case example of male therapist and male patient both engaged in competitive running (not exercise during therapy), at times against each other. Altshul commented: "Our involvement in running was invariably turned to therapeutic advantage. . . . Such disparate affects and motivations as competitiveness and longing to be close could be expressed in the language—not to mention the activity—of running" (p. 54). Male-female pairs may operate on the assumption that the man has or is supposed to have greater skill and power. Particular tension can arise if the woman is in fact faster, stronger, or has better endurance. Female-female pairs are likely to be somewhat more idiosyncratic in their approach, based on individual sport history.

Exercising together creates many opportunities to attend to body image, body awareness, and issues of sexuality. Exercise appears to be associated with increases in self-efficacy, self-concept, self-esteem, and body image (Berger & McInman, 1993). Major psychotherapeutic benefits may accrue, as illustrated in the case examples below, with survivors of sexual abuse. Yet because of shifts from the typical psychotherapeutic strictures, it is critical that the therapist review and monitor clients' perceptions of the experience.

> **Exercise during therapy would be a pain in the ass for me. I show an aggressive side when I am involved in physical activity that is not suitable for client contact. Besides, this is a private experience for me. In some ways it is better than what others report as religion is to them.**
>
> **50-year-old male psychologist**

Gender pairing and sexuality enter the everyday details as well. Sport clothes, as compared with street clothes, reveal and emphasize the body. The informality and camaraderie surrounding exercise can influence the therapeutic frame. There is a natural tendency to appraise the other's physique, whether out of attraction or comparison. After a run, people typically begin peeling off excess layers of clothing, even if it be only running shoes. Locker room culture uses different rules and meanings than does the therapy office. Opinion varies as to whether this needs to be a concern. Johnsgard (1989) commented that patients can handle seeing their therapists in sweats and sweaty. However, the suggestiveness and intimacy of changed breathing patterns and alterations of dress may in some situations override the benefits.

The excitement of a joint project—as when verbal therapy is going especially well—can lead to a sense of synergy. Yet it is important to acknowledge that this very excitement can result in a certain preciousness for the client and therapist who exercise together. In running therapy, the typical hubris of runners can be compounded by a recognition that this is a unique form of therapy; the client has a special connection with the therapist—a shared interest or passion. The slippery slope of sexual suggestiveness or exploitation (Brodsky, 1986; Rutter, 1986) has all the more potential to develop in this circumstance. Once again, therapist and client gender, sexual orientation, and client history are important elements. Particularly when working with clients with a history of incest, the therapist must be cognizant of the evocation of the secret, special, physical patterns of relating associated with this abuse (Herman, 1992).

Walking During Therapy

Perhaps because it is so simple and common, walking may be considered the aspirin of exercise. When exercise is recommended, walking is probably the safest and most frequently proposed. Walking is the exercise of choice for physicians encouraging their patients to exercise, weight loss support groups (e.g., Weight Watchers), and medically managed weight loss programs. Few studies, however, have examined the effectiveness of walking on mental health.

When therapists suggest exercise to their clients, they, too, often recommend walking. Walking meets Berger's (1994) taxonomy criteria of exercise that is rhythmic, continuous, requires steady breathing, is not dependent on the development of a complex skill, and is non-competitive.

Anecdotally at least, it appears that if exercise is used during therapy, it is most likely to be walking. Walking is safe even for the obese, it can be used as a method to ameliorate anxiety in vivo, client and therapist can maintain a dialogue while walking together, the logistics are fairly simple and straightforward, and it may serve as the base for developing other exercise habits (Sime, 1996). Likewise, because it is so ordinary, walking with a client may be fairly straightforward and potentially less complicating than running.

Alice entered therapy with acute symptoms of major depression, panic disorder, vivid posttraumatic stress disorder (PTSD), and morbid obesity. Food consumption had been a long-standing and primary method of managing the other three symptom clusters. She had a history of severe and unremitting physical and verbal abuse by her mother as well as violent sexual abuse by her brother.

Initially, I suggested exercise because of its biochemical capacity to decrease anxiety and depression. Exercise, I explained to Alice, was a powerful method for controlling panic and alleviating depression. Regular exercise also would be the most effective, least threatening, means for beginning true weight loss—one of her primary objectives. Subsequently, the distraction of exercise gave her better access to imagery around trauma resolution.

The use of a stationary bicycle and decreased bingeing resulted in a 20 pound weight loss over a 10-month period. This weight loss was sufficient to ease a chronic foot problem, and Alice began walking occasionally. In the midst of a very difficult time during which she confronted both her mother and brother about her childhood experiences, she also suggested a few times that we walk for part of the therapy hour, which we did.

With the resolution of her history of severe physical and sexual abuse, Alice began feeling comfortable enough in her own body to undertake more intense weight reduction efforts. In addition to dietary management and regular attendance at a community weight management support group, she began walking on a systematic, daily basis. At this time, at her suggestion, we began to walk routinely while conducting therapy. Initially, we walked for about 20 minutes of the session, although within 2 months we were walking the entire session. We covered varying terrain—hills and flats—and continued through winter snow and by summer gardens—about 2½ miles each time. Alice increased exercise at home to about 5 miles a day, 5 to 6 days a week. Just as with stationary bicycling, walking now had a number of purposes: to sustain the weight loss, to regulate mood, and to create time and means to think through issues.

Alice commented: "Pondering difficulties while I'm fully engaged in physical activity allows me to visualize new approaches. I feel 100% of me is free to engage my mind in solutions and possibilities. My mind feels less cluttered, my thinking is unencumbered by negativity."

Alice's beliefs about herself and exercise changed. She described herself as craving exercise. She was excited to have muscle definition. "Movement is such a gift," she commented one day.

As her clothing changed from overblouses to wearing a skirt with a waist band, we were able to discuss the meaning of having a waist, of being feminine. As a woman beginning to develop shape and definition, she recognized changes in her perception of herself with a figure: instead of being a victim, she could see herself as powerful and strong.

For the most part, the content of the therapy session was the same as it would have been in the office. Yet there were differences, too, metaphoric opportunities that could be enacted. Alice used the symbolism of her newfound strengths. As we began one session, she remarked: "Let's do hills today. I have stressful things to talk about." Typically, we commented on flower gardens we passed, and the meaning of those comments provided a subtext. At the termination of therapy, Alice said: "I really did understand the symbolism of all those flowers we looked at; the growth and the beauty and the things in their season."

Running During Therapy

Although running during therapy was described by a few practitioners with great enthusiasm in the 1980s, even anecdotal reports no longer are appearing, with the exception of an article I wrote in 1994. That case is described here briefly.

Polly was a 32-year-old, lesbian doctoral student, teaching at a small college. As an adolescent, she informed the police of her father's 12-year history of sexual assault on her, and he was arrested, tried, found guilty, and incarcerated.

As is true of many incest survivors, Polly entered psychotherapy with a residue of effects from her early history

(Courtois, 1988; Gelinas, 1983; Hays, 1985, 1987; Herman, 1992). Relational concerns included passivity and activity, boundary diffusion, relationships with authority figures, and problems with intimacy. Often emotionally flooded, she had difficulty integrating affect, cognition, and action. She experienced violent, terrifying nightmares, chronic disorganization of time and money, and significant lapses in recollection of her history.

Polly entered one session in such agitation that she could not sit still. She began pacing the room. It was a beautiful New England fall day, and I knew that Polly regularly engaged in various forms of strenuous exercise with a number of friends, so I suggested that we continue therapy while walking. She was immensely relieved at the suggestion, and we pursued the content of the session while we walked about a mile. Polly commented favorably on the walk. Intrigued by the seeming helpfulness of movement to her therapeutic process, I asked whether she would be interested in trying a session while running. She was immediately enthusiastic.

Over the next year, we ran during most of the subsequent sessions, maintaining a pace that allowed us to talk. With a standard circuit of about 3 miles, there was enough time when we returned to the office for us to draw conclusions, summarize, and resolve any remaining issues.

Polly, who at times was reduced to inarticulate tears in the office, was able while running to experience, express, and understand her emotion. In a number of sessions, the increased capacity to observe as well as experience herself was strikingly evident. Although this improvement may have been in part a function of length of treatment, the treatment medium also played a significant role.

During one session, we discussed major tensions around her mother's role in not protecting Polly from abuse by her father. Polly began running faster and with greater intensity. I suggested that she sprint, and she did so for a quarter mile. I, who usually slowed my pace slightly to accommodate hers, was unable to keep up. Later, she commented: "I ran as fast as I could—letting the anger out with each step. I felt as if I was releasing myself from a tangle of emotional obligation to my mother. I felt drained and yet stronger. I'm not one for yelling; this seemed like the same kind of release someone else might get from yelling at the top of their lungs."

Given Polly's comfort with physical activity and her overwhelming anxiety in the office, running therapy helped her sustain the balance of emotional safety and risk taking that underlies successful change. That running therapy worked so well with her underscores the important conjunction of a number of factors: the naturalness and timing of the suggestion, the client's history of exercise as a means of connection, exercise as a part of her core identity, and comparable pacing, stamina, and zeal for running.

III | THE PSYCHOLOGICAL BENEFITS OF EXERCISE WITH SPECIFIC POPULATIONS

Overcoming Inertia: 7
Exercise and Depression

D epression, one of the most common complaints among adults seeking psychotherapy, is nonetheless underdiagnosed, undertreated, and costly (Too few people, 1997). It has been estimated that clinical depression strikes approximately one fifth of Americans at some point in their lives and that only 27% of cases receive adequate care (Rich, 1997). The direct and indirect costs, financial as well as emotional, are staggering. Including treatment, premature death, absenteeism, and lost productivity, the cost may be as high as $43 billion annually (Too few people, 1997). Treatment recommendations typically are for some variation of psychotherapy or somatic intervention (antidepressant medication, electro-convulsive therapy, or light therapy) alone or in combination (American Psychiatric Association, 1993).

Treatments have their own costs. An American Psychiatric Association survey of appointment and prescription rates found the following changes over a 9-year period: In 1985, 32.73 million visits to the doctor (5.1% of all visits) resulted in prescriptions of psychotropic medication. By 1993–94, psychotropic medication was prescribed during 45.64 million appointments (6.5% of all visits) (Pincus et al., 1998). Further, the number of office visits as a result of depression doubled between 1988 and 1994. Antidepressants now account for the greatest number of psychotropic drugs prescribed in the United States.

Medication for depression has a number of uncomfortable potential side effects. Among these are dizziness, sedation, anticholinergic effects, weight changes, sexual dysfunction, neurological side effects, cardiovascular effects, insomnia, and anxiety (American Psychiatric Association, 1993). In the era of selective serotonin reuptake inhibitors (SSRIs) and a swing of the pendulum toward biological explanations and treatments, one somatic approach that appears to be effective yet entirely out of the current experimental mainstream is the use of exercise, alone or in combination with psychotherapy or medication.

The following case illustrates the use of exercise in treating depression, as well as the individualized meaning of exercise and the experience of subjective vs. objective levels of fitness (Martinsen, 1990; Mondin et al., 1996).

> Prematurely wizened, 42-year-old Prentice shuffled carefully into my office. Since his daughter's illness at age 10 and subsequent death from leukemia 5 years before, he had been incapacitated by back pain. It now prevented him from moving with any comfort. Fear of greater pain exacerbated his bodily rigidity and heightened his panic as he contemplated negotiating an icy winter. The previous summer, an orthopedist and a physical therapist had treated him, and he had been able to walk a few miles a day. Discouraged when his back went out again, Prentice felt emotionally and physically near paralysis.
>
> I reviewed Prentice's case with his physician. Discouraged by his patient's frequent hospitalizations, the physician was treating him primarily with antidepressant medication. There appeared no physiological basis for his pain.
>
> For several reasons, exercise seemed an essential aspect of his treatment. In the past, Prentice had in part defined himself through athletics. Throughout his school years, he played various sports. As an adult, he was a fierce racquetball competitor. Now, his debilitation served as a constant reminder that he was not himself. Becoming active again would help him regain a sense of connection to his earlier self and support his development toward a feeling of wholeness. Furthermore, tangible progress could signal hope and a reason for living, in contrast to his current regression toward immobilization. Increased muscular flexibility would decrease the risk of injury or the exacerbation of his back problems as a consequence of muscular rigidity. Additionally, Prentice recognized that when he was more active he felt physically better—and better about himself. Lastly, being active and out in the world would afford Prentice the opportunity for social contact, from which he had been withdrawing.
>
> Prentice declared that walking would be therapeutic for him, and we discussed opportunities and options available to him. It was not until well into treatment that Prentice revealed that he had been physically active all along: on instruction of his physical therapist, Prentice had used an exercise bicycle twice a day for the past number of months. The bicycle had, no doubt, been effective in preventing loss of muscle tone and maintaining some physical flexibility. It apparently had had no effect on his state of mind.

Our brief discussion concerning exercise bolstered Prentice' intentions. By our third interview, he had decided to rejoin his racquetball club. Though he longed for fresh air, he ruled out the natural setting because he disliked winter weather and feared the icy footing. The racquetball club had an indoor track that he could use for walking.

At our fourth interview, Prentice clearly moved with greater ease and his mood was less tinged with hostility and truculence. He had begun walking at the club, and had also started walking around his office building. He enjoyed the social atmosphere of the club. He wondered about consulting with the physical therapist within a few months to determine his readiness to use the club's Nautilus equipment. Prentice described himself as already feeling and acting considerably more friendly toward coworkers.

If he were going to give up the somatic symbolization of his pain, it had become clear that Prentice would need to further work through the unresolved grief over the loss of his daughter as well as other significant familial tragedies. Strikingly, it was during the fourth interview—just after he had begun his walking program—that Prentice spontaneously began to actively grieve his daughter's death. With increasing emotion, he related her last moments and funeral. He offered to bring in pictures of her. Each week thereafter, he would walk casually into the office, comment that he was feeling fine, report on how frequently he had walked, and then spend the remaining time talking and crying about his daughter, dredging up memories long carefully stored away. The rigidity with which he contained his emotions loosened as his bodily stiffness diminished.

A markedly controlling and defensive man, Prentice not only determined the content of each session, but also rarely accepted any direct advice or suggestion. Thus, any specific exercise prescription I might have made would have been met with hostile rejection. Support for and encouragement of his exercise plan were the most active interventions that could be made, and were essential. Additionally, pain management techniques helped Prentice decrease his dependence on medication and increase his sense of efficacy.

In an unspoken way, as a runner I served as role model for Prentice with regard to exercise. True to his rigid and sardonic manner, he teased about the danger and stupidity of running (and, by not so subtle implication, of runners) in contrast to his more healthful form of exercise. Yet, tacitly expressed was the sense of community among people valuing exercise.

Depression and Exercise

In what seems a nearly apocryphal story, aerobics guru Kenneth Cooper (as recounted by Sime, 1996) told of a man with heart disease who was depressed:

[He] was so despondent that he wanted to die. Because his heart was weak, he thought the best way to commit suicide without embarrassing his family was to run around the block as fast as he could until he killed himself. After several futile attempts at causing a fatal heart attack in this manner, he discovered to his surprise that he began to feel better and eventually chose to live instead of to die. (p. 176)

Of all the clinical issues for which exercise has been recommended, depression has been most frequently and commonly studied (Martinsen, 1990). Reviewed here are some conclusions from a meta-analysis of the effect of exercise on depression, followed by descriptions of some specific studies.

A total of 80 studies with 290 effect sizes, dating primarily from the 1980s, were reviewed using a liberal definition of depression, and including both aerobic and anaerobic exercise (North, McCullagh, & Tran, 1990). Major findings included the following:

- Exercise was a beneficial antidepressant both immediately and over the long term.
- Although exercise decreased depression among all populations studied, it was most effective in decreasing depression for those most physically or psychologically unhealthy at the start of the exercise program.
- Although exercise significantly decreased depression across all age categories, the older the participants (age range was 11 to 55), the greater the decrease in depression with exercise.
- Regardless of gender, exercise was equally effective as an antidepressant.
- The most frequent forms of exercise used were walking and jogging.
- All modes of exercise examined, anaerobic as well as aerobic, were effective to at least some degree.
- The greater the length of the exercise program and the larger the total number of exercise sessions, the greater the decrease in depression with exercise.
- The most effective antidepressant effect occurred with the combination of exercise and psychotherapy.

> On a day-to-day basis, regular exercise helps my cognitive processes. I think, plan, and execute tasks better. I enjoy the benefits of better health, improved stamina, and being able to do things that others my age may not. It also is a major stress release. (My wife has remarked on more than one occasion when I am ruminating over an irritation, "Don't you need to go for a run?") It helps me put things in perspective and balance. There also is a major social component of portions of exercise, particularly the cycling that I do with friends. Long, slow bike rides in the country nurture the spiritual aspects within me, and the long slow distance runs are times that I do some of my best planning and perspective checks.
>
> **47-year-old male psychologist**

In reviewing and summarizing some of these same studies, Johnsgard (1989) concluded: "The magnitude of change which results from exercise therapy by itself is as great as that associated with a variety of standard group and individual psychotherapies, some of which, in turn, have been shown to be as effective as antidepressant drug therapy" (p. 135). He suggested that it is important in future research on exercise and depression to select patients carefully, not only based on the severity of depression, but also etiology (endogenous vs. exogenous depression).

Comparison of Exercise and Psychotherapy for Depression

If exercise functions as an antidepressant, how does it compare with psychotherapy? In a classic study by John Greist and others at the University of Wisconsin, 28 patients presenting for treatment at an outpatient psychiatric clinic with a diagnosis of unipolar depressive disorder were randomly assigned to running therapy, time-limited individual psychotherapy, or time-unlimited psychotherapy (Greist and colleagues (1979). The running condition participants showed improvement in depression equivalent to the two psychotherapy conditions at the end of 10 weeks of therapy, and at 1- and 3-month follow ups.

> **I have often thought that it would be helpful to walk with certain clients + talk as we walked—get them moving, shake things up a little.**
>
> **43-year-old male psychologist**

Because of some methodological difficulties with the first study, Klein et al. (1985) assigned 74 participants meeting the criterion for unipolar depression randomly to four conditions:

1. running therapy: individual meeting with therapist in two 45-minute sessions each week. There was minimal talking, and that which occurred focused on individualizing the run-walk plan, breathing, and the participant's experiences with independent running between sessions;
2. meditation-relaxation to provide a contrast treatment that would incorporate some of the body awareness and mastery aspects of running without the aerobic component;
3. weekly 2-hour group sessions including breathing and yoga-based stretching exercises designed to help participants

focus and control breathing while achieving a deep state of relaxation;

4. semistructured group therapy with elements of interpersonal and cognitive therapy for 2 hours a week over 12 weeks.

Participants in each treatment condition showed decreased depression at termination. The outcomes were somewhat better for running and meditation than for the group methods, even over 9-month follow up. There were few differential or specific treatment effects, and the treatments were considered to be generally of equal effectiveness.

Exercise With Psychiatric Inpatients

Discussion of the use of exercise with the chronically mentally ill is reserved for chapter 12. Here, findings from a number of international studies on depression are described. It is perhaps significant that there appears to be no research on the use of exercise with acutely depressed inpatients performed in the United States. Norwegian psychiatrist Egil Martinsen is one of the few to have conducted experimental studies of patients undergoing psychiatric hospitalization for nonpsychotic mental disorder, most commonly unipolar depression. Martinsen commented (1990) that in general, depressed patients, and hospitalized patients, tend to be sedentary. (One should note, however, that cultural factors are evident as well: Of the patients he studied, 23% exercised regularly prior to admission, in comparison with twice that number in the general adult Norwegian population. Figures in the United States would be considerably lower on both counts.)

Although it is in certain cases a somewhat arbitrary demarcation, distinction is made here between patients hospitalized for depression and those who are severely and chronically mentally ill. In one investigation, 49 inpatients diagnosed with major depression were randomly assigned to 1 hour of aerobic exercise (training group) or 3 hours of occupational and milieu therapy (control) in addition to one to two sessions of individual psychotherapy per week. After 6–9 weeks, significant reduction in Beck Depression Inventory scores and therapist ratings of depression were noted for both groups. However, the reductions in the training group were significantly greater than in the control group.

In another study, Martinsen, Hoffart, and Solberg (1989) compared 99 inpatients with major depression, dysthymia, or depression not otherwise specified (NOS) with regard to the effect of aerobic vs. anaerobic exercise on depression. In contrast to some earlier findings, they noted that both groups experienced significant reductions in depression, whether or not their aerobic power had increased.

One of Martinsen's most intriguing findings has been the result of patient comparisons of the usefulness of exercise with other forms of treatment. "Patients evaluated physical fitness training as the most important element in the comprehensive treatment programmes. It was ranked above traditional forms of therapy: psychotherapy, milieu therapy and medication" (Martinsen, 1990, p. 386). This information contrasts with a generally held belief that patients do not like strenuous exercise. It also is significant in regard to prediction of exercise maintenance. Martinsen reported that more than half the patients continued to exercise one year after termination of the formal training program (1990).

In a study of 18 nonpsychotic, nonmedicated inpatients (mean age of 34), Dutch psychiatrist Rudi Bosscher (1993) compared walking and running with mixed forms of anaerobic exercise. Although the depression scores remained high, the running group showed significant improvement on depression, whereas patients engaged in mixed physical exercise did not improve significantly on any measure. Self-esteem increased over time for both treatment conditions. Bosscher comments that the improvement in self-esteem but not depression for the mixed group suggests that "a boost of self-esteem may be a necessary but insufficient prerequisite for a change in depression" (p. 179).

There are no definitive studies of the effect of physical activity on psychotic depression or bipolar disorder (Martinsen & Morgan, 1997). Martinsen and Morgan (1997) do, however, describe three avid male runners, all on lithium, who attempted to taper the medication and replace it with daily running. All relapsed and needed to resume lithium within a year. In another brief case description, a 23-year-old man with frequent brief hospitalizations for psychotic episodes experienced various side effects from major tranquilizers. Following a regimen of running, weight lifting, judo, and eclectic psychotherapy, there were no further psychotic episodes or hospitalizations, and the patient showed substantial emotional and physical gains (Gleser & Brown, 1988).

Psychotropic Medication and Exercise

At age 43, Melissa, a slight, angular, and bitter woman sought psychotherapy because of chronic dissatisfaction with herself, her marriage, and her work. She had been running for 5 years, and claimed that only during and shortly after her daily runs did she feel any alleviation of her gloom. Despite attempts at various forms of individual psychotherapy, Melissa, herself a mental health professional, found fault with them all and continued to feel unrelievedly bad about herself. Following a medication assessment, Melissa responded to antidepressant medication with decreased anger but no overall alleviation of her depression. Although not optimally effective, it appeared that the most useful treatment for her was the combination of medication and exercise. With her agreement, psychotherapy was discontinued.

In marked contrast to the various studies that have been conducted comparing the effectiveness of psychotherapy and medication in treating depression, there have to date been no formal experiments comparing exercise with medication, let alone combinations or a three-way comparison. Minimal information is available concerning the use of exercise for patients who are currently taking psychotropic medication. Some of Martinsen's patients have been taking tricyclic antidepressant medication. In one study, he found that those who were medicated had similar reductions in depression scores to those who were not medicated, whereas there was a trend in another study toward better outcome for those on medication and exercising (1990).

Pragmatically, in addition to problems associated with initially low fitness levels among this population, there may be increased management issues for those on medication, caused by such medication side effects as dryness of mouth, drowsiness, and increased heart rate. Martinsen (1990) suggests keeping exercise intensity low while adjusting medication dosage. Exercise intensity should be increased only once the patient has reached a steady medication state.

Perhaps most surprising, in light of the frequent prescription of selective serotonin reuptake inhibitors (SSRIs), there is currently no information available concerning exercise among patients using this class of medication. Martinsen and Stanghelle (1997) devoted a full chapter to drug therapy and physical activity yet included only one paragraph about SSRIs. They hypothesized that since SSRIs tend to have fewer adverse effects than the classical tricyclic medications, there are likely to be even fewer problems with their use than with previous medications (Martinsen & Stanghelle, 1997).

Women, Depression, and Exercise

Regardless of race, education, occupation, nationality, willingness to seek help or report symptoms, twice as many women as men experience unipolar depression (McGrath, Keita, Strickland, & Russo, 1990). At any given time, in the United States 2–3% of men and 4–9% of women suffer from depression (Kahn & Fawcett, 1993). Although the lifetime risk for major depressive disorder has been estimated as ranging from 5–12% in men, it is estimated at 10–25% for women (Martinsen & Morgan, 1997). A biopsychosocial perspective on depression suggests that social, economic, biological, and emotional factors all contribute to this international statistic. Likewise, a sociocultural perspective recognizes that women are much less likely than men to consider exercise under any circumstances, let alone when they are depressed and experiencing symptomatic low energy and decreased sense of initiative. Further, a focus on depressed feelings and passivity rather than mastery and action among depressed women (McGrath et al., 1990) would predict less likelihood of exercise. It has been noted that women receive 70% of the prescriptions for antidepressant medication and, further, that there is a high risk of improper diagnosis and misuse of prescription drug use among women (McGrath et al., 1990). For all of these reasons, then, women may be a subpopulation within the depressed population for whom exercise is especially important, albeit particularly challenging.

> Although she discovered the helpfulness of running as an antidote to depression during college, 26-year-old Annette has also been in and out of therapy over a number of years, and has used psychotropic medication. On a low maintenance dose of Prozac (10 mg every other day), she still experienced considerable situational depression. Encouraged to monitor her level of depression using a 10-point subjective mood scale, she noted a mood improvement of at least 2 points on the scale each day after she ran. Monitoring herself internally, she was aware that this mood elevation persisted throughout the day.
>
> Annette realized how authentically helpful the running was when, one particularly difficult day, the score was 2 points lower after the run. She had awakened that morning feeling even more depressed than usual. On this day, she felt so low that the physical effort of running depleted her further, physically and affectively. Recognizing that she had registered a decrease on this particular day, she felt increased confidence that this simple subjective measure was providing an accurate reading of her mental state.

In a controlled experiment on the relationship between exercise and depression, McCann and Holmes (1984) randomly assigned 43 depressed undergraduate women to an aerobic exercise, relaxation, or no treatment condition. Women in the exercise condition developed improved aerobic capacity, and level of depression decreased significantly more than among women in the other two conditions. Roth and Holmes (cited in Holmes, 1993) subsequently tested whether aer-

> Clients usually respond initially with enthusiasm (to the suggestion of exercise). Then they have to confront the inner limits and feelings of what they deserve or don't deserve, in terms of feeling good about themselves or taking time for themselves. What sounds like a quick fix becomes the beginning of a process of self-examination and discovery.
>
> **44-year-old female psychologist**

obic fitness could be useful in preventing the onset of depression following prolonged psychological stress. In a 2 × 2, life stress by level of fitness design, college students who were not fit and had experienced high life stress showed depression in post-testing 9 weeks later, whereas those with low stress, regardless of fitness, and those who were highly fit, did not develop depression. Holmes suggests that aerobic fitness may serve a prophylactic function, as well as having the potential to moderate the relationship between stress and depression.

Practitioner Recommendations

Because someone who is depressed may be fairly inactive, the importance of obtaining health clearance before encouraging exercise cannot be overemphasized. Receiving support from his or her health care provider may also serve as further reinforcement for the client to undertake this change in behavior.

Since depression often includes components of psychic immobilization and motor retardation, people who are depressed may not be especially venturesome or interested in making use of their bodies. Specific subjective rating scales can help a client develop a concrete awareness of the acute effects of exercise in alleviating depression. For example, a client may keep a 1–10 rating of mood before and after exercise, such as was used by Annette. There is good empirical support for this clinical suggestion. Using the Profile of Mood States, McGowan and Pierce (1991) found that the mood of college students enrolled in activity classes improved from before to after session.

Once clients have become accustomed to exercise, they may be encouraged to keep track of the length of time for symptom relief. Not only will this draw attention to the effectiveness of exercise but it also will serve as an antidote to the belief that the depression is unremitting.

In addition to acute effects (see Glossary), the length of time that one has been exercising correlates with decrease in depression. Thus, assisting the client in persisting with exercise is critically important. If a client does not note the type of acute changes described above, the therapist may focus initially on those changes that are occurring. The therapist may draw the client's attention more toward improvements in cardiovascular functioning, physical strength, or self-care. The therapist can help the client recognize that the mental effects may emerge more gradually.

Since continued exercise following treatment has been associated with prior adult use of exercise (Martinsen, 1990), it is useful to help patients recall their prior exercise involvement. Those without such a prior history may need more support and assistance in planning an exercise program.

People who are depressed are often likely to distort information through all-or-nothing thinking, overgeneralizing, and magnification. When embarking on exercise behavior, it is important to help the patient set small, incremental and realistic goals, both in terms of physical conditioning and as a model of attending to the positive aspects of behavior.

Although these suggestions are couched in behavioral terms, it is generally important to understand the person's thoughts, feelings, and attributions around exercise. Idiosyncratic explanations, catastrophizing, and negative self-attributions all are hallmarks of depression. These assumptions and beliefs can be used as examples with the client in understanding typical patterns of thought, particularly in regard to new experiences.

Depression often involves social isolation. An exercise program involving others may therefore be especially helpful, although this may be a long-term, rather than an immediate, goal. Even if a person is exercising with others, it is important to review and potentially help the client revise their mental messages. Invidious comparisons do nothing to help a client feel better.

When working with someone who is taking psychotropic medication, titration of exercise is recommended. Martinsen's suggestion of low initial exercise intensity is the only guideline that currently exists.

For those who have been exercising for a long time, habituation may result in a less powerful exercise effect at times of increased depression. During such periods, it may be helpful to alter some aspect of the FIT (see Glossary). Although there may be individual differences as to which aspect to shift, my experience has been that increased intensity often serves an acute function. Clients also may report a resurgence of positive mood over a few week period following increases in frequency or duration.

Calm in Motion:
Exercise for Anxiety

8

Along with depression, anxiety disorders are among the most prevalent forms of mental illness and the most frequently treated. It has been estimated that in the United States approximately 7.3% of the adult population warrants treatment for anxiety (Raglin, 1997). Further, there is considerable comorbidity between major depression and anxiety. In various studies, 44–91% of patients with panic disorder also were diagnosed with major depression (Clayton, 1990). As with depression, the use of exercise can be a self-directed, inexpensive alternative or adjunct method of treatment.

Forty-seven-year-old Gordon, a part-time coach with whose team I had previously consulted, called on self-referral. He described a history of panic attacks, current high levels of anxiety, and a desire for increased relaxation and self-confidence.

During intake, he elaborated: "I don't feel in charge of my life. I have a real problem with unknowns. I am physically tense much of the time. I don't enjoy myself enough. I feel easily threatened by things, and take criticism the wrong way. I'm too sensitive."

The eldest of three, Gordon had grown up in an alcoholic household in which he experienced his father as highly critical, dissatisfied, and punitive with him. He described, for example, an incident during which his father deliberately ran over his bicycle because he had left it in the driveway. His mother was always there, but passive and self-absorbed. His maternal grandmother was the one unconditionally nurturing figure in his life.

Following a brief hospitalization in his late teens for acute depression, no subsequent problematic history occurred until 2 years prior to this contact. At that time, Gordon experienced an intense and prolonged panic attack while driving. Prior to that, over a fairly short span of time, five close relatives, including his maternal grandmother, died. Convinced that he was having a heart attack, he went to the hospital, where he was diagnosed with panic disorder. Since then, he had experienced mild to moderate anxiety attacks on a daily basis. He lived in pervasive dread of a return of the Big One. Tingling in his fingers and lightheadedness occurred frequently throughout each day.

A doting parent himself, Gordon explained that his youngest child had just left for college, and he and his wife had recently moved to a new community, at some distance from former neighbors and friends. He described having a great relationship with his wife, although he added that she was not sympathetic and seemed to have little interest in his thoughts or feelings. He said they had few friends locally. "There's nobody I can really talk to in my life."

He had seen a therapist twice previously, once after the initial panic attack, and again a year later. She taught him some "techniques to hold the attacks at bay," which he found of immediate help but which did not allay his underlying dread. He had been using Xanax for the panic attacks. Prozac had been prescribed for intermittent depression, although he currently was not using it. His physician seemed comfortable with his continuing to use Xanax PRN indefinitely.

During that first session, I taught Gordon deep breathing techniques (see Glossary) and encouraged him to use these methods four times a day initially. I also tried to normalize the tingling fingers and light-headedness by naming these symptoms as hyperventilation. Reframing, I suggested that he could use his awareness of these symptoms as a cue to practice deep breathing and potentially decrease the attacks or their intensity.

Although he had a long history of physical activity, Gordon currently was not exercising at all. The previous winter, he had walked 2 miles daily. I would have encouraged him to resume walking, as it had been a part of his earlier routine, but I was concerned that the low intensity might not have much immediate impact on his considerable level of anxiety. Hoping to address that anxiety through tension regulation, I suggested that he explore taking a yoga class to reinforce diaphragmatic breathing and develop new movement skills.

Self-reliant, Gordon took a number of significant actions over the next few sessions:

1. He reported using the deep breathing regularly—not as frequently as I had recommended, but at least two to three times a day.
2. He did not follow up the suggestion of yoga, but instead enrolled in a local exercise club and began working out.

3. Impulsively, he discontinued Xanax entirely for a week, and although he seemed to tolerate the physiological changes, his anticipatory anxiety remained high. We discussed a much more gradual taper of the medication, as he built up a sense of confidence in his own capacity to manage his anxiety.

4. He began to have casual conversations with colleagues at work and recognized that he felt somewhat less emotionally isolated.

5. He began paying more attention to and acting on some of his own interests. For instance, he went to a jazz concert. While there, he became aware that he was not feeling claustrophobic. Characteristically, he then began worrying—about his lack of anxiety.

Although Gordon continued to be unwilling to systematically track his negative mental messages and positive reframes, discussion of mental processes increased his awareness of those negative messages. He used this awareness, however, to berate himself for being so negative. There were ways in which his self-punitiveness was even more debilitating than fear of recurrence of panic attacks. Using the analogy of his skills as a positive and supportive coach of an athletic team, we discussed ways he could go about being a more constructive coach to himself.

By the fourth session, Gordon reported systematically using exercise after work as a method of daily stress management. He enjoyed having a sense of reclaiming his body, seeing it as powerful and capable while still continuing to view his physical self as frail and unpredictable. He also remained anxious about his competence in the work setting. He experienced a high level of stress in particular on Mondays, the beginning of the work week. I suggested he consider exercising before work on Mondays.

With limited managed care coverage, therapy sessions with Gordon were spaced out over time, and discontinued before he was fully symptom free. He still occasionally experienced light-headedness or tingling and numbness in his hands or feet. He had learned the cognitive skills of redirecting attention and decreasing his catastrophizing. Yet given the number of times we had discussed deep breathing and its effectiveness for him as both preventive of and antidote to hyperventilation, it surprised me that this was not yet a part of his automatic repertoire.

By termination, Gordon had discontinued all medications for 2 weeks. He was still experiencing some residual physiological and psychological symptoms of anxiety, but was markedly less fearful about another impending major panic attack. He continued to have some self-doubts about whether he was really capable of being medication free, and so he continued to carry a few pills with him, just in case. He seemed very clear that in order to lower his general arousal level, he would need to do it physiologically—through exercise or meditation and relaxation.

The interpretation of research on exercise in relation to anxiety is confounded by various linguistic, conceptual, and methodological issues. The term *anxiety* at times refers to increased levels of physiological arousal, stress response, tension, state (momentary) vs. trait (persistent tendency toward) anxiety, or clinical levels of anxiety. Further, much of the research in relation to anxiety has relied on self-reported measures that may or may not bear a relationship to physiological measures of arousal. Likewise, measures of anxiety have either assessed response to acute bouts of exercise (see Glossary), that is, how one responds immediately to the effect of the exercise, or chronic exercise (see Glossary), that is, changes over time in relation to exercise. Nonetheless, and although there have been some inconsistent findings, in general it appears that both acute and chronic physical activity are associated with decreases in anxiety both for people with normal levels of anxiety and for people with elevated anxiety levels (Long & Stavel, 1995; Petruzello & Landers, 1994; Raglin, 1997). The decrease in anxiety may last for 2 to 4 hours at a time.

> The combination of listening to music while exercising increases my optimism.
>
> 41-year-old female psychologist

Some research has focused specifically on levels of intensity needed to moderate the effects of anxiety. In a study of the relationship between exercise and optimism, participants who engaged in aerobic or a combination of aerobic and anaerobic exercise (see Glossary) experienced significantly lower levels of trait anxiety than those engaged only in anaerobic exercise (Kavussanu & McAuley, 1995). Although earlier research suggested that exercise intensity should be at least moderate, studies with hospitalized patients reported positive results with aerobic, low intensity, or strength training exercise, even when there was not significant physiological improvement. There is some equivocation about whether high-intensity exercise results in an increase in anxiety. So many differences between studies exist, including training level, degree of psychological impairment, type of exercise, perceived exertion, and timing of postexercise assessment, that it is not possible to draw definitive conclusions concerning optimal generic intensity levels for the alleviation of anxiety (Raglin, 1997).

In a comparison of community residents with clinically significant anxiety, Steptoe, Moses, Edwards, and Mathews (1993) examined whether intensity of aerobic training reduces physiological stress response. "Moderate aerobic training led to increases in physical fitness and greater improvements in ratings of tension, depression, confusion and ability to cope with stress than did the attention-placebo training" (p. 116f.). Those in the moderate training group experienced increased confidence in their ability to cope with stress, even though subjective ratings of mood or coping ability did not correlate with changes in physiological stress reactivity. Steptoe and colleagues concluded that although aerobic training might not lead directly to lowered physiological stress responsivity, changes in cognitive appraisal and coping helped alter that physiological reaction. "Moderate aerobic training leads to significant reductions in anxiety, depression and mental confusion, together with improved perceived coping ability" (p. 125).

Exercise to Inhibit Panic Disorder or Agoraphobia

A few early studies sounded an alarm by suggesting that panic attacks could be precipitated by vigorous exercise. Continuing reference to these methodologically questionable studies may have dampened interest and limited subsequent research on the use of exercise for clinical anxiety (Raglin, 1997). A more recent study of 16 panic patients matched with 15 normal controls found only one instance in which a patient panicked during bicycle ergometry (Stein et al., 1992). Stein and colleagues concluded that panic attacks were not driven either by exercise-induced distress or by exercise-related metabolic changes.

> With a 30-year history of agoraphobia and panic disorder, 61-year-old Hilda sought treatment after she found herself increasingly constricted in her activities. An initial focus on methods and instances of not panicking helped her begin to feel in some control of her responses. She had been walking—and enjoying it—regularly for some years but now added this to her conscious armamentarium of coping behaviors. Over a 6-month period, she kept a daily chart of panic attacks and the use of coping behaviors. As the intensity of her anxiety decreased, she became slightly more venturesome. Over the next year and a half, we met once a month for supportive therapy.
>
> Toward the end of that time, I asked her to write down her thoughts on why exercise was important to her. She started by describing her walking route in great detail, focusing on particular gardens she passed, places she had worked, her beloved church, smells and mental associations, her own long history in this neighborhood, and connections with other people. At times, friends joined her or she paused to chat. She

During the work week, initially my mind usually roams with work thoughts, dilemmas, or schedules. I have found that if I start out at whatever pace feels comfortable for my body and mind that day, these thoughts run their course in short order. I then begin thinking about the rhythm of my heart + lungs + muscles, the feel of the sweat, and mini-goals for the workout. My mind turns to enjoying the technical aspects—improving the quality of my skating, improving my running form, lengthening my stride, increasing cadence, and so on. I notice a lot through my sensory experience of the world around me, too—smells, sounds, trees, birds, and wind. I usually take routes that have the least traffic and most natural environment. On running days, it is almost always off-road. I enjoy the meditative state of exercise, with thoughts nowhere in particular or roaming freely.

34-year-old female social worker

enjoyed surveying ways that she and others had improved the community. "When I walk it's a time to be with me. It not only helps me physically to shape up but it's a peace of mind time. It seems to help me focus. It makes me breathe deep, it helps to strengthen my legs, my arms, my whole body, and especially my mind. I wonder if people who see me on my route, smiling, know how much this means to me. No, they probably don't know why I'm smiling—but I know and that's all that matters."

Panic disordered or panic attack patients may feel uncomfortable—anxious about inducing a panic attack—with increased heart rate as a result of exercise (Clayton, 1990). Yet it is possible to use those sensations to reframe symptom meaning, using a method of interoceptive exposure (Barlow & Cerny, 1988). Twenty-five years ago, Orwin (1973) developed a novel treatment method for psychiatric inpatients or day patients who had a long history of agoraphobia or panic disorder. Patients were assigned to run from a safe setting to a designated place where anxiety symptoms typically occurred. Arriving with autonomic arousal that could be reattributed to their physiological state, and repeating this action, patients experienced rapid symptom remission along with a strong sense of mastery. Orwin described a housebound 45-year-old patient with a 13-year panic disorder history. She responded rapidly to this treatment, and Orwin concluded: "Not only was she completely free from all symptoms but she was very confident because she felt that by her own effort she would have the ability to overcome any tendency to relapse" (1973, p. 177). Rapid, forceful action, the method generally used to control anxiety, was co-opted for a different purpose. The autonomic excitation involved in exertion competed with and inhibited the anxiety, and any autonomic components of anxiety could be reframed cognitively as part of the body's response to physical exercise.

Physical Activity During Therapy to Help Contain Anxiety

Even if the primary diagnosis is not anxiety or panic disorder, at times clients present in session with considerable anxiety. In some instances, and in certain therapies, it is useful for the therapist not to intervene in the presence of this manifestation. At other times, a therapist may explore the meaning of the anxiety or make use of it as an occasion for the client to practice anxiety management techniques. Alternatively, there are times when as a therapist I have experienced the therapy session as being at an impasse: therapist and client sit, facing each other, the client becoming more withdrawn, immobilized, and silent. Anxiety may be at the heart of the stalemate. On occasion, at those moments I have suggested that we move outside the office to continue our session. Running therapy with a client, described more fully in chapter 6, began in just such a way (Hays, 1994b). For another client, Shana, an attempt was made to help a session become more productive:

> Referred by her couples therapist for individual therapy, 27-year-old Shana, herself a therapist, was brittle and self-conscious throughout our sessions, apparently continually second guessing herself as she focused on the shame of her history and behavior. "I feel dysfunctional and damaged," she commented. After 4 months of sessions, she was, if anything, even more constricted than earlier, shutting down affectively, leaving sessions early, canceling appointments at the last minute, unable to think of what to talk about. She self-censored, sure that I would see how messed up she was.
>
> Rather than continuing to hope that we could work through or ride out the tension, I suggested during the 11th session that we try walking as we spoke. Although there was initially much silence, as we walked she finally began to talk about a prior painful therapy experience.
>
> Shana was already exercising regularly and finding that it decreased her irritability. This in-session walk was not designed to encourage exercise per se as much as to manage anxiety so that Shana would be able to do the work of therapy. We used this method one more time, again when she was extremely tense, and again, she was more verbal, although still ambivalent about therapy.

In addition to recommending walk-talk therapy as a method of supporting exercise initiation (Sime, 1996), Sime (personal communication, February 11, 1998) also has encouraged walking during therapy as a

> When I exercise, my thinking is more relaxed (vs. pressured), more like acknowledging what I have to do rather than getting anxious about what I have to do.
>
> **25-year-old female doctoral student**

means to break a client's anxious impasse. Similarly, Kabat-Zinn (1990) described a client at the University of Massachusetts Medical Center's stress reduction program whose already high level of somatic anxiety increased markedly when she attempted to engage in the stillness of mindfulness training. It was only through walking meditation that she could begin learning methods for stress reduction.

Practitioner Recommendations

Exercise as a method of tension release for somatic expressions of anxiety has an immediate intuitive appeal. Although it may be a somewhat larger leap to understand its effectiveness with cognitively experienced anxiety, clients are likely to notice reductions in mental as well as physical manifestations, and both acute and chronic anxiety, through the use of exercise. As with exercise for depression, clients' attention can be drawn to these effects. Encouraging clients to rate their level of tension before and after exercise may help them understand the effectiveness of this tool for anxiety reduction.

Exercise methods that necessitate, incorporate, or emphasize diaphragmatic breathing may be especially useful for clients with anxiety, as this regulated breathing will itself serve to decrease physiological levels of arousal. Thus, hatha yoga, which typically includes a component of relaxation training, is recommended. Likewise, aerobic activities impel diaphragmatic breathing.

For clients who are ruminative, forms of exercise that involve a modicum of skill acquisition or attention may prove useful in distracting them from internal processes. Alternatively, methods of redirecting attention can be incorporated into the regular rhythm of repetitive activities.

Clients dwelling on anxious thoughts during exercise may be encouraged to use either associative or dissociative strategies of thinking (see Glossary). For example, clients who swim could be encouraged to redirect their attention to the sensation of pulling their arms through water, or those who run could focus on the depth of their breathing. This may best be accomplished by changing the intensity of the exercise. Alternatively, dissociative methods could involve developing and repeating an affirmation in rhythm to one's activity.

There is no information on whether clients with obsessive-compulsive disorder may be at increased risk to exercise compulsively. It may be possible to explore this risk with the client before embarking on an exercise program and to use the exercise as an experiment at handling anxiety in a new way. Lesyk offered a poignant and frustrating case history in which the client's driven focus on exercise reinforced a dysfunctional family system (1998, pp. 47–48).

Following Orwin's lead, it may be useful to consider running as a method of interoceptive exposure within a cognitive-behavioral protocol for patients with panic disorder. As with other methods of flooding, clients can learn to reinterpret physiological signs of arousal.

The varied findings from research suggest that regardless of the intensity of exercise, individual prescription that incorporates the client's own history, skills, and interests is most likely to be successful.

Staying Sane:

Exercise and Stress Management, Self-Esteem, and Mastery

9

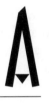s with depression and anxiety, considerable research has been conducted concerning the effectiveness of exercise in the management of stress, and exercise is typically a standard component of suggestions for stress management. Much of the available research has been conducted on convenience samples of (nonclinical) college students (Berger, 1994). The findings from these studies translate most directly to people experiencing situational crises, or the worried well. Although stress is not per se a diagnosable problem or syndrome, clients are commonly seen for issues in which stress is a component. Situational stressors may exacerbate already tenuous functioning, or an accumulation of stresses may become overwhelming.

28-year-old Donna was referred by a family member a month after the death of her beloved younger brother in a motorcycle accident. "I can't believe they did this to me—the one person in the whole world I totally trusted and loved," she cried. Donna was socially isolated, undereducated, psychologically naive, and frustrated by low-paying and unstimulating in-home childcare.

To alleviate stress, it might have made sense to recommend exercise. However, the pragmatic issues of lack of time, limited finances, and lack of interest suggested that superimposing such an expectation on her would have seemed at best irrelevant. Donna did mention, however, that she was on a darts league with her husband. One of my initial suggestions was that when she was throwing darts, she could mentally aim at "them"—the nameless external force that had taken her brother from her.

Stress is so ubiquitous in our language and our lives that it is important that I clarify the interlocking linguistic and definitional network. Following that, I will consider the short- and long-term benefits of exercise in stress management and relevant types of exercise.

Definitional Issues, Mediating Factors, and Interaction With Exercise

A number of interacting concepts are described here, relating to stress, coping, stress management, arousal, self-esteem, and body image. Recognizing these interrelationships allows for a more complete understanding and the potential to intervene at various points.

To be alive is to experience stressors. Hans Selye, who coined the terms *eustress* and *distress* to describe both the positive and negative aspects of stress, suggested that finding one's optimal stress level allows one to live life most fully (Selye, 1975). However, the term *stress* commonly refers specifically to the experience of distress, the perceived discrepancy between one's capacities and the behavior or response necessary to cope with a perceived stressor (Berger, 1994). That meaning is used here.

> I exercised regularly as a child and in high school, quit in college, and didn't start again until I was about 30. I got started again mostly for social reasons. Health is most important now, both physical and emotional.
>
> **51-year-old female psychologist**

Variables that moderate the stress-illness relationship include coping style, health care practices, and social support. Specifically, physical exercise may serve as a buffer against the negative impact of high levels of stress. Support for this assertion comes from a number of sources: anecdotal reports of the stress-reducing properties of exercise, controlled laboratory studies, and systematic observation of the tempering effects of naturally occurring stressful life events (Brown & Siegel, 1988; Rejeski, Thompson, Brubaker, & Miller, 1992).

Stress implies heightened levels of both physiological and psychological arousal. Thayer (Thayer, Newman, & McClain, 1994) has developed a theory of mood that focuses on the dimensions and interactions of energy and tension. "Mood is assumed to be closely associated with central states of general bodily arousal with conscious components of energy (vs. tiredness) and tension (vs. calmness)" (p. 911). The most negative mood states are those combining both low energy and high tension. Optimal levels, alternatively, are the result of activities that raise energetic arousal, reduce tense arousal, or affect both systems simultaneously. And exercise serves to regulate exactly these functions. "Moderate exercise has proved to be one of the most effective mood-regulating behaviors, probably because its primary mood effect is enhanced energy, but a secondary effect is reduced tension" (p. 912). Further, since skeletal-muscular tension is a component of tense arousal, "behaviors that affect this bodily system would be important in mood regulation" (p. 912). More colloquially, one can move a muscle and change a mood.

Thayer also suggests that there is a holistic interaction between cardiovascular, skeletal-muscular, and cognitive aspects of the self and positive and negative mood. This implies that change in one system will likely affect other systems simultaneously. Preferred levels of energy and tension vary under different conditions, as well as by personality. Type A people may prefer a moderate degree of both tension and energy.

Self-esteem, a multicomponent construct, relates to capacity to function with adaptability within society and feel in control of one's life. Low self-esteem is related to depression and psychopathology (Sonstroem, 1997). Self-esteem is often described as an evaluative component of one's more global self-concept. Self-concept is considered "an individual's overall awareness of self in regard to physical attributes, personal characteristics, social identities, and/or behaviors" (Horn & Claytor, 1993, p. 312). Self-esteem, on the other hand, "refers to the individual's evaluation of or affective reaction to these attributes or characteristics . . . the value the individual places on those self-perceptions (i.e., degree of satisfaction with what he or she is)" (Horn & Claytor, 1993, p. 312). Self-esteem reflects one's global life adjustment and overall sense of well-being (Sonstroem, 1997).

The relationship between exercise and self-esteem is intricate but important. A simplistic implied syllogism of the exercise-self-esteem relationship may include the following elements: exercise makes you feel good; feeling good increases your self-esteem; therefore, exercise improves your self-esteem.

Needless to say, human beings are more complex—and less linear—than this reasoning suggests. There are various ways in which self-esteem and exercise interact. Sonstroem (1997) has suggested that physical exercise and the resultant physical fitness leads to increased physical self-concept (an estimation of one's physical abilities), a component of total self-esteem, which then leads to increased interest in physical exercise, in a repetitive, positive loop.

Self-esteem is related to both one's sense of skill and self-enhancement. Describing a "bidirectional rubric," Sonstroem pointed out that "experiences in the environment can impact self-esteem (skill development hypothesis), and self-esteem can in turn influence experiences in the environment (self-enhancement hypothesis)" (1997, p. 129). As one becomes more skilled physically, there is an increase in self-esteem. Likewise, as one feels better about one's physical skill, performance skill increases. It appears that "higher levels of self-regard following exercise intervention are based on perceptions of improvement or other program or score factors rather than on fitness improvement itself" (p. 131). Gains in self-esteem through exercise are greater for those with initially lower self-esteem scores, as well as those with lower fitness who value an increase in some aspect of fitness or skill. Further, it appears that these increases in self-esteem are relatively long-lasting.

Other aspects of self-esteem involve a sense of competence, mastery, or self-sufficiency, and a broadened or increased sense of identity. Johnsgard (1989) suggested that internal self-statements may become, for instance, "No doctors. No pills. I did it. I know how. I could do it again" (p. 50), or a sense that in addition to whatever else I may be, I am a physically active person. Exercise becomes more important, and the self becomes more important.

Body image is another of the self-esteem–exercise interactions. Dissatisfaction with body image is correlated with low self-esteem, insecurity, and depression, regardless of gender (Rejeski & Thompson, 1993). However, there are complex mediating variables in relation to gender. Men and women, across various studies, differ in what is important to them. Whereas strength, physical condition, and increased weight are important to men, women tend to want to be thinner, whether or not that goal is objectively warranted.

Immediate and Long-Term Effects on Coping and Self-Esteem

Exercise may influence two different aspects of coping. First, exercise can be an emotion-focused coping response, helping to regulate emotional or physiological reactions to a stressor event by inducing relaxation, changing mood, or serving a distracting function. It may have acute or short-term impact by helping to reduce emotional or physiological reactions. Chronic or long-term effects, when regular exercise is maintained, include improved cardiovascular function, which in turn increases physiological stamina and energy. Improved body image may result from alterations in body shape as a function of redistribution of weight and changes in muscle definition. Second, exercise may affect one's primary appraisal process, and thus be a resource for preventive coping. Internal or external demands may be appraised as less threatening or harmful if the exercising person has a sense of confidence that exercising will help reduce bodily tension or enhance mood. Over time, the exercising person may have an increased self-efficacy for mastering challenging tasks, "if their acquired knowledge from regular exercise was stored in long-term memory as self-schemata relating to mastery, control, and self-regulation" (Long, 1993, p. 350).

In an experiment involving low to moderately physically fit women, Rejeski, Thompson, Brubaker, and Miller (1992) created psychosocial stressors (Stroop test and an impromptu public speech) both in the absence of and following a bout of 40 min of aerobic exercise. In the exercise condition, the participants' blood pressure reactivity was dampened, and the frequency and intensity of anxiety-related thoughts was diminished. Although pointing to the potential for exercise as an alternative to pharmacological methods, Rejeski and colleagues recognized that further research is needed to determine the length of time following exercise that physiological and psychological responses continue to be attenuated. Additionally, there continue to be questions of the dose-response relationship.

> Charlotte, 48, was diagnosed with bipolar disorder and effectively treated with a combination of psychotherapy and Tegretol (200 mg. t.i.d.). Two years later, I was following her once a month essentially for support and occasional "course correction": She still had a tendency to speak and act impulsively, especially within her immediate family, in an interpersonally chaos-producing manner. At this time, her father, with whom she had an enmeshed attachment, was diagnosed with a rapidly metastasizing cancer. Charlotte was devastated by his degree of illness and her impending loss. She had by then been taking regular daily walks "to clear my mind" for a while. Throughout the last stages of her father's illness, she began using her breaks at work to walk: She would go two times around the building at break and three times at lunch. She commented, "This is what's keeping me sane." Supporting this constructive means of coping, I also encouraged her to be systematic: She could use a part of the walks for deep breathing and calming, and part for regrouping and planning.

Kavussanu and McAuley (1995) found general optimism among those exercising regularly. Because they conducted a cross-sectional study, the directionality of this relationship could not be determined. In another of those synergistic loops, Kavussanu and McAuley suggested that exercise may decrease trait anxious apprehension. A sense of mastery through activity may increase one's positive outlook. Alternatively, a positive sense of self may lead one to engage in health-promoting behaviors, in turn resulting in a sense of well-being. Long-term as well as short-term effects, then, are posited.

Using an experience sampling method, Gauvin, Rejeski, and Norris (1996) found that acute vigorous physical activity among women accustomed to exercise was associated with significant improvements in affect and feeling states, particularly feelings of revitalization, positive affect, positive engagement, and tranquility. Measuring negative affect separately, they observed a statistically significant, although less powerful, decrease in negative affect. The greatest positive change in mood occurred for those who felt worst before the physical activity. Gauvin and colleagues concluded that

> acute physical activity is not systematically associated with feeling better; rather, it is related to more beneficial changes in mood if mood is somewhat lower before activity. . . . The potential of acute physical activity in maintaining psychological well-being may lie in its efficacy to modify affect and feeling states when they are at undesirable levels while leaving them relatively unchanged when they are normal or positive. (p. 395)

> During my internship, I used running as a major strategy for coping with the stress of ending a relationship. I have maintained an active exercise schedule ever since. When I started private practice, I intentionally started playing competitive volleyball as an "anchor" to my schedule. In practice it is too seductive to think "I'll just see one more person and make X dollars more." The boundary between work and personal time is so easily blurred, that knowing I had a different activity that I would hold as a priority was crucial. The social aspect has become an integral part of our family life.
>
> **47-year-old male psychologist**

Exercise and Stress Management

Exercise, a standard tool of stress management, at times appears to have a greater impact on psychological than physical measures of stress. The effect of exercise may be more psychological than physiological for those without serious psychopathology (Berger, 1994), or it may be that there are not yet equally effective methods of measuring the physiological effects. Examining whether aerobic training reduces physiological stress response, Steptoe, Moses, Edwards, and Mathews (1993) found that "moderate aerobic training led to increases in physical fitness and greater improvements in ratings of tension, depression, confusion and ability to cope with stress than did the attention-placebo training" (p. 116f.). Moderate aerobic training did not decrease physiological stress responsivity; however, changes in cognitive appraisal and coping may serve as a moderating variable to help alter physiological stress responsivity. "Participants in the moderate training group also felt greater confidence in their ability to cope with stress, indicated by the increases in reported 'coping assets'" (p. 122).

Exercise is a practical and multifunctional method of stress management. It often requires little equipment, can be done at home, is inexpensive, and does not have undesirable side effects (Berger, 1986). It affects one's physiology as well as mind, increasing the stroke volume of the heart, reducing blood pressure, increasing high-density lipoproteins, increasing muscular strength and endurance, improving physical appearance, resulting in loss of fat tissue, and, therefore, promoting desirable weight without dietary restriction, and helping to retard or reverse osteoporosis.

Yet although exercise is an effective tool in stress management, experimental comparisons with randomized designs suggest that it is not necessarily more effective than other stress-management techniques. Meditation, the relaxation response, progressive relaxation, and stress inoculation training all can be used to alleviate stress (Bahrke & Morgan, 1978; Berger, Friedman, & Eaton, 1988; Long, 1985; Long & Haney, 1988). Furthermore, these techniques needn't stand alone. The combination of cognitive (mind to body) techniques with somatic (body to mind) techniques is especially intriguing (Berger, 1986). Exercise can be combined with other techniques for stress management. Benson (1984) suggested that this works best when meditation is combined with

> I dedicated one midday, midweek run recently to my friend Joe who died last fall. I had a really good piano lesson the day before in which a new piece I had written was well-received by my instructor, and he encouraged me to title it. I decided to call it "Where's Joe?" On the run, I allowed myself to go over a number of the pieces I've worked on over the last year and improvise in my head, as I'm not yet able to do very successfully in vivo. It was a wonderful, creative, poignant time which went well beyond the issue of my subjective experience of being mired in loss to a healing time of remembering, grieving, and creating.
>
> **51-year-old male**
> **licensed pastoral psychotherapist**

rhythmic, smooth, repetitive, noncompetitive individual activities that do not demand either complete attention or unusual alertness, in other words, those aerobic activities with the characteristics of Berger's (1994) taxonomy. With running, Benson suggests focusing on one's breath, saying "in" and "out" silently to oneself as one inhales and exhales, or using one's footfalls to a count. Likewise, with swimming, one can focus on breathing or use the arm motion to think "left" and "right." A practical book, *Jogging the Mind* (Green, 1995), gives detailed instruction on combining aerobic exercise with meditation.

Practitioner Recommendations

When recommending exercise for stress management, the practitioner has many options:

- The client may use exercise as a distractor from tension, a time out.
- The client may use exercise as a time to work creatively on problems or their solutions.
- The client may use exercise to regulate social distance. In handling stress, people's desire for social contact varies. For some people, part of the stress-reducing quality of exercise is the camaraderie of the team or the locker room. Others feel that exercising alone is often one of the few moments they can legitimately have to themselves.
- Before and after measures of tension or tiredness can reinforce the helpfulness of exercise in stress reduction.
- Combined exercise and meditative techniques may further enhance the stress-reducing properties of exercise.

A tension headache, knotted stomach, or momentary distractibility may actually be one of the few opportunities people have to fully recognize the unity and physiological and psychological interaction of mind and body (Berger, 1994), even if most people would not describe themselves as fully enjoying this recognition and interaction. However, in pointing to these negative effects, it is also possible to attend to the positive interactions of mind and body through exercise and movement.

The more stress a person is experiencing, the more positive effect can be anticipated through exercise. As with other syndromes and symptoms, clients may find it very useful to note subjective ratings of stress in relation to exercise.

I am a terrible technical swimmer. When I swim, I focus almost exclusively on technique, monitoring my actions and movements and trying to count the laps. When I cycle with a pack, I am exquisitely focused on the events around me, the distance and interrelations between the other riders. On our long social (conversation pace) rides, we are liable to talk about anything. If there are just two of us—either my wife or my training partner—we use the time to talk about issues in our lives. We've used those rides to deal with deaths, job changes, and births of babies. Track workouts are back focusing again on technique.

My long, slow distance runs are a personal treasure. While I occasionally run with others, my real preference is to do it solo. I use that time as a major opportunity for reflection and planning—similar to hypnotic trance. It is a flowing process between both convergent and divergent thinking. Although I may be able to duplicate the process in nonexercise settings, the distractions and demands of other contexts would serve as major obstacles.

47-year-old male psychologist
(triathloner)

Simultaneous ratings also can prove of diagnostic and treatment utility. Comparison of somatic vs. cognitive effects of exercise can be instructive. A client who reports "I was still just as depressed, but I felt less tense after exercising" may need additional suggestions and supports regarding the depressive aspects of her or his problems.

As with many other aspects of self-efficacy, exercise programs designed to enhance self-esteem need to emphasize success experiences, feelings of increased physical competence, and goal attainment. Although the therapist can hope that these are the conclusions the client will draw, directing attention to positive attributions and outcomes increases the likelihood of these effects. An overall sense of mastery may be increased by generalizing certain key personal characteristics from the exercise experience, such as persistence and optimism.

The positive effects of exercise in stress management will be increased if a person anticipates and attributes changes to exercise and mastery. Johnsgard (1989) comments: "When we begin to exercise every day, insist that an hour of each day belongs to ourselves exclusively, and tell others that they will have to somehow adjust their needs and expectations to allow us our exercise period, we're making a strong statement about ourselves: 'My running is important. My time is important. My needs are important. I am important'" (p. 50).

Loss and Gain: 10
Exercise and Eating

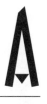 long with its myriad of physical and psychological benefits and connections, exercise has some specific eating- and weight-related effects and interactions. The possible moderating effect of exercise in relation to eating and weight with regard to physical and emotional status is also of interest. Exercise can help regulate appetite, alter food preferences, and reinforce healthier eating habits. Further, "exercise not only offers potential for weight reduction, but also helps ameliorate certain of the risk factors linked to obesity, such as heart disease" (Heil & Henschen, 1996, p. 241). Additionally, the mediating effect of increased self-efficacy can in turn boost self-confidence and consequently may improve thought and mood regarding weight management (Rodin, 1992). At the same time, pathological interactions between exercise and weight, especially at the lower end of the scale, merit careful review.

In this chapter, I will describe a variety of links between exercise and eating, both those that are additive or synergistic as well as those that are troubling. Specifically, I will address the interaction of gender and weight, dieting, and exercise; and issues around exercise with various clinical populations (clients with obesity, bulimia nervosa, and anorexia nervosa).

Gender, Weight, Diet, and Exercise

In our society, food, eating, weight, and exercise have gender-specific components and meanings. It is normative for women to be preoccupied about food, weight, and body (Bordo, 1993). "For an overwhelming number of women in our society, being a woman means feeling too fat" (Rodin, Silberstein, & Striegel-Moore, 1984, p. 267). Women's bodies have been objectified for centuries. "Women's bodies have always and everywhere been perceived as unfinished, in want of carving, perforating, incising, refining, and realignment" (Rodin, 1992, p. 24). Women's bodies become a "mobile billboard for their owner's brilliance, energy, and savvy" (p. 26).

> I've become less obsessive about exercise and weight control. It seems like there are no reasons I could think of to not enjoy movement and my personal strength and to check out my limits in various fields of sport.
>
> **44-year-old female psychologist**

Women bond and compete around issues of thinness and physical attractiveness. Focus on food and weight is a means of connection, whether through the media (e.g., women's magazines) or more personally (a friend's struggle with her latest diet). At the same time, these areas "may be the chief and most wholeheartedly sanctioned competitive domains in which women are encouraged to contend with each other" (Rodin, Silberstein, & Striegel-Moore, 1984, p. 290). The downside of functioning in a relational manner is that women live life comparing themselves to one another—as well as comparing themselves internally to an unattainable idealized, fantasy woman engendered by the media.

As women in our society move into previously male-dominated professions, they may experience competing needs to both minimize and retain their female status. Since physically attractive women are perceived as more feminine, women can have their cake and eat it, as it were, by being simultaneously powerful and attractive (i.e., thin; Rodin, 1992).

Additional gender differences occur in regard to weight preoccupation, weight loss, and maintenance of that loss. As if it were a diabolical plot, women are at a number of sociocultural and physiological disadvantages regarding an issue that tends to have much more meaning for them. In general, men are less encumbered by the sociocultural web surrounding the interaction of food, eating, nurturance, and weight. Men typically have more lean body mass and less body fat than women, and since lean tissue is more metabolically active than fat, tend to have a higher metabolic rate (Thompson & Sherman, 1993). With higher resting metabolic rates, men require more calories to sustain general functioning. Since they have not dieted as frequently as women—women are twice as likely as men to report that they are dieting to lose weight (Stephenson, Levy, Sass, & McGarvey, 1987)—men's bodies have not developed the metabolic slowdown that results from weight cycling (Rodin, 1992; Striegel-Moore, Silberstein, & Rodin, 1986). Thus, they tend to be able to lose weight and maintain weight loss more easily. And men more easily turn to exercise for weight control than do women.

While men and women share in the likelihood of obesity, women are more heavily stigmatized in our society for being overweight. Further, the eating disorders of restriction, that is, bulimia and anorexia, are preponderantly gender-specific disorders. These disorders may be the extreme version of women's "normative" concerns around weight (Rodin, Silberstein, & Striegel-Moore, 1984).

Even though in this chapter I primarily address issues relative to female experience, men certainly have concerns around weight, body image and self-esteem, and exercise. For example, overweight men participating in either weight reduction or aerobic conditioning in a long-term program experienced positive changes in MMPI scores. In contrast, depression scores for control participants increased (Koeppl et al., 1992). Nonetheless, the particularly complex interaction of socialization and social context with both weight and exercise for women suggests, for the most part, numerous gender differences in focus and approach.

Obesity and Exercise

Defiantly, 40-year-old Joyce exclaimed, "I don't want to diet any more!" She was startled when I responded with equal fervor: "Great!" A much-silenced mother of three who worked in her husband's business, she had entered therapy with tearfulness, fatigue, low self-esteem, and fuming irritability. Being overweight added to her sense of shame and social isolation.

After some discussion, Joyce decided to walk with her neighbor and their children to and from the school bus stop on a daily basis. She developed the courage to tell her (surprised) husband of her wretched unhappiness, which in turn emboldened her to talk with a friend and begin to feel less alone with her pain. She commented that this was the first time she had ever started to lose weight by developing a regular pattern of exercise prior to the initiation of dieting. Although she wanted to lose weight, she was now really clear that she did not want to go on a diet.

We discussed the virtues of lifestyle and habit change rather than quick, backfiring fixes. Joyce was intrigued by referral to a registered dietitian who conducted a group on healthy weight management. Empowered by her now-predictable walking pattern, she transferred that sense of self-efficacy to the potential for weight loss.

DISCUSSION

Approximately 34 million adults in the United States are obese. Of those, 20 million are women. Another 20 million women are overweight or perceive themselves to be so (Kirschenbaum, 1992). Inactivity, it has been suggested, contributes more to the maintenance of obesity than does overeating (Heil & Henschen, 1996). The interaction of inactivity and obesity becomes compounded. "As weight increases activity decreases" (Heil & Henschen, 1996, p. 241).

Conversely, exercise and weight loss are associated in a number of ways. Most obvious is the sheer balancing act of caloric intake vs. expenditure. Exercise uses up more calories than does sitting still. There are additional benefits as well. When one decreases caloric intake through dieting, metabolism is suppressed, with a concomitant slowdown in the body's functioning. Exercise, in contrast, serves to increase the body's resting metabolic rate. Further, the body continues at a higher metabolic rate for a time after exercise, thus maintaining more efficient functioning. Moderate exercise tends to decrease, rather than increase, appetite, and may change food preferences toward more balanced eating (Foreyt & Goodrick, 1992; Summers & Wolstat, 1984). Since muscle burns more calories than does fat, increase in muscle mass (through exercise) results in greater caloric loss. In contrast to other methods of weight loss, exercise attacks body fat rather than lean body tissue. Exercise appears to be the one method for lowering an individual's *set point*, the homeostatic weight regulation mechanism that tends to keep people at a stable weight (Kirschenbaum, 1994).

A number of positive psychological effects of exercise in relation to weight loss also occur. In addition to general improvements in mood associated with exercise, people often experience an increased feeling of control as well as a sense of self-efficacy. As with Joyce, there may be a sense that "if I can take charge of my exercising self, I can make choices about what and when I eat." Further, exercise may have a profound impact on both body awareness and hunger awareness (Sheehan, 1978), each an important component of weight loss.

Although weight loss is a challenging process, by far the more difficult stage is the maintenance of that loss. Perhaps even more dramatic than the role played by exercise in weight loss is its role during maintenance. Contrary to many people's implicit theories, changing one's exercise patterns is at least as important as changing one's eating habits in order to attain permanent weight control (Kirschenbaum, 1992). What kind of and how much exercise is necessary is still not entirely clear. And the reinforcing effect of persistence per se may be a major contributing factor. Nonetheless, one of the most accurate predictors of weight loss maintenance is the maintenance of exercise (Brownell, 1994; Kirschenbaum, 1994). "Increasing exercise may be the single most important thing an individual can do to lose weight and keep it off" (Kirschenbaum, 1992, p. 83).

PRACTITIONER RECOMMENDATIONS

Especially with overweight clients, it is important to differentiate the role of therapist from that of physician. Overweight clients should be strongly encouraged to review any physical limitations with their health care provider before embarking on any particular strenuous activity. Even if clients feel uncomfortable initiating such discussion, most health care providers will be very supportive of any interest shown in increasing physical activity.

With obese clients, it is important to attend very carefully to the client's stage of change regarding exercise behavior. Obese clients tend to have had numerous encounters with the prescription of exercise. They therefore may bring to such discussion a variety of negative experiences and injunctions. Initially, they may be externally, rather than internally, motivated around this issue.

Clients may be actively aware of the general benefits of exercise, but may need assistance in developing specific personal values and beliefs regarding physical self-efficacy. Recognizing the range of possible kinds of exercise, appreciating the social and pleasurable aspects of moving one's body, and developing graduated goals with systematic periodic review, all can increase the likelihood of exercise adherence (Goodman, Bergandi, Morgan, & Lewis, 1996).

Exercise adherence among the obese may be compromised as a function of body or physique anxiety (Heil & Henschen, 1996). An overweight client may experience a tremendous sense of shame about her body. Anything that makes her feel more visible may be resisted on those grounds alone. Thus, for example, although the prescription of swimming may be exactly the right suggestion in terms of a client's history, skill, enjoyment, convenience, and so on, the thought of exposing her body to others in this way initially may be daunting to her. She may be responsive to joint problem solving: Her primary discomfort may be the anticipation of nakedness in the locker room rather than the actuality of wearing a bathing suit or being in the water. Helping her find ways to have sufficient privacy may allay her anxiety.

Monitoring progress in a journal can provide information and self-support. Along with keeping a log of food eaten, or fat calories, or pounds lost, keeping a detailed record of the amount and kind of exercise helps the client understand patterns. A weekly graph can further summarize and reinforce changes in activity level.

Weight distribution changes with exercise (Brownell, 1994; Kirschenbaum, 1994). I often encourage clients to measure themselves before beginning a regular pattern of exercise. This provides an alternate measure to that derived from The Scale, and may be the area of change most quickly noted. As body weight becomes redistributed, clothes start to fit differently and a person becomes and begins to appear leaner.

The satisfaction of movement can translate metaphorically as well. As a person becomes accustomed to exercise, this activity can come to be experienced as a different way of feeding oneself, nourishing the body and clearing the mind.

Bulimia: The Vicious Cycle

A long and lanky 29-year-old woman with a 15-year history of disregulated eating (past anorexia and current bulimia), Erica tackled exercise as she did everything else—chaotically and with a vengeance. Running and aerobics were performed with determination but without plan, excesses following droughts. Driving herself physically was gratifying to this woman who felt little satisfaction with most of her life. Exercise was yet another venue to punish herself while ostensibly doing the right thing.

As she developed greater self-acceptance, she also gradually let go of bingeing and purging. Exercise took on a predictable pattern, one that allowed for pleasure with activity for its own sake.

DISCUSSION

The "natural" bodily patterns and rhythms of eating can become disregulated in a variety of ways. Some are cyclical and set into action a perpetual motion machine. Binge eating without purging results in weight gain. The cycle of bingeing and restriction can become self-perpetuating: The typical pattern involves a cycle of food restriction, followed by overeating, with resulting guilt and shame in turn leading to efforts to rid oneself of the effects of the action. Subsequent restriction maintains the vicious cycle. Although purgatives (vomiting or laxatives) are more common methods, a number of people use high-intensity aerobic exercise for self-punitive weight control.

We all overeat some of the time, or eat when we are not especially hungry. As described in the previous section, additionally, exercise is an effective component of weight loss. And many people are motivated to exercise in part for weight control. Likewise, there are many social supports for being thin and for exercise (Rodin, 1992). The issue of bulimic exercise, then, is more a matter of degree than kind. It is a matter of intention and affect (Walsh & Garner, 1997). This is not to diminish the reality of bulimia, which can be physically damaging and is experienced as extremely distressing and out of control. Instead, it is intended to point to the distinguishing character of bulimic exercise. Rather than experiencing exercise as energizing and pleasurable, exercise is meted out in a desperate attempt to right the scales. Obligatory intensity diminishes the possible psychological benefits.

PRACTITIONER RECOMMENDATIONS

As with other forms of purging, the issue for bulimic clients who use exercise as a self-perpetuating attempt at balancing or undoing the effects of binges is to help the client figuratively or even literally stand still. Exercise in this context is understood to be but one of the protective, homeostatic, and defensive processes that may be used in bulimia.

Accurate indexes of excessive exercise have not been developed (Walsh & Garner, 1997). Nonetheless, clients may assess their behavior through keeping track of exercise patterns. Charts, such as Fairburn (1995) has developed, which include space for vomiting, laxatives, or diuretics, can be adapted to include a column for obligatory exercise.

In addition to behavioral measures, one can address the cognitive and affective elements of exercise as a pathological weight control mechanism. For example, a client may come to understand the meaning of exercise by developing a chart of her automatic thoughts and rational responses regarding eating and exercise. Alternatively, a journal-type "dialogue" between oneself and exercise can assist in understanding the role of exercise in perpetuating the bulimic behavior. As the internal battle

> Potentially a person could become obsessed with exercise as a means to the idealized body shape and use it as the purge part of bulimia. But I have not had this happen with the clients to whom I have recommended exercise, even though I have worked with women for whom bulimia was a presenting issue or at least part of the presenting issue.
>
> **44-year-old female psychologist**

involving bingeing, punishing, and deprivation becomes more visible and obvious to her, the client can feel more control over ways she can intervene in her own behavior. By clarifying, recognizing, and naming her concerns, she can address and resolve them.

As with other disorders of eating, the goal, ultimately, is to assist the client in regaining a sense of food as food, weight as only one part of a person's self-definition, eating as related to actual physiological hunger, and exercise as part of connecting with one's entire—including bodily—self.

Anorexia and Ascetic Exercise

The enticement of bulimia lies in its homeostatic intent. It is a balancing act. In contrast, the drive toward power through nothingness forms the seductive core of anorexia. As Bruch (1978) commented a generation ago, anorexia is a "relentless pursuit of thinness." Experienced as a companion, a means, or a slave master, exercise can be swept up in that relentless pursuit. To be able to run endless hours signals the triumph of will over body. Excessive exercise has been implicated as a possible indicator of subsequent poor prognosis in anorexia recovery (Casper & Jabine, 1996).

> An exquisite, stylishly dressed, petite young woman with flowing blond hair, 30-year-old Diana presented herself for therapy because of food preoccupation and a method of weight control that had almost entirely shut out her social life. "My whole life is targeted on diet and exercise," she commented. After a full day of work, she regularly rode her exercise bicycle for 3 hours, ending up exhausted and drained. She had neither energy nor time for her new marriage, and did not allow space for the development of friendships or other activities in her new location.
>
> Diana reported a history of disordered eating and weight control for at least the past 11 years, including laxative abuse, some abortive attempts at vomiting, and days-long starvation. She recognized that she was trying to control both anxiety and depression through weight and exercise management. She felt caught in the cycle, out of control of her rumination and behavior. She had attended couples therapy briefly, but dropped out because it interfered with her workouts.
>
> Initially eager to attend a therapy group for women with bulimia or anorexia, she dropped out after one session. She felt anxious about her desire to compete for thinness through

increased exercise, and was unable to contain her anxiety enough to deal with it within the group.

Diana returned to individual therapy 1½ years later: She was about to be discharged from an inpatient unit, having been hospitalized for postpartum depression and panic. Along with considerable support and assistance from various community agencies and frequent contact with the psychiatrist who was medicating her, I worked with her on developing skills and a sense of capacity to care for her infant and, in the process, come to a different understanding about her capacity to nurture herself. She developed a few tenuous friendships with women she met in a postpartum exercise class. Although clearly at continued risk for further difficulty, she was also more aware of and responsive to her own needs and their positive resolution.

DISCUSSION

In a number of studies designed to tease out the interaction of eating disorders, obsessive characteristics, and exercise, Davis and colleagues (e.g., Davis et al., 1995) have compared anorexic inpatients with corresponding community samples, focusing in particular on the relative frequency and duration of exercise. They suggested that an interacting triad of related factors—exercise, obsessive compulsiveness, and dieting—appears to be related to the pathogenesis of eating disorders. "The relationships among physical activity, starvation, and obsessive compulsiveness tend to be reciprocal and dynamic" (Davis et al., 1995, p. 974), potentiating each other in a destructive, self-perpetuating loop.

The interaction of excessive or compulsive exercise and body satisfaction is one that has been subject to considerable recent study. However, varying measurement issues make it difficult to draw definitive conclusions at this time (e.g., Brewerton, Stellefson, Hibbs, Hodges, & Cochrane, 1995; Davis & Fox, 1993).

Bordo (1993) and Yates (1991) have each described a kind of asceticism, not unlike the medieval saints and martyrs, as a central feature of anorexia. This austerity focuses on purification, will, discipline, the conquest of desire, aspiration toward an ideal, and transcendence of the body. Extremes of exercise can fit naturally into this pattern. And although there have been a number of criticisms of Yates' research (Brownell & Rodin, 1992), the metaphoric similarities certainly are compelling. Whether it is causally connected or coincidental, both committed exercisers and anorexics tend to be perfectionistic, achievement oriented, highly motivated, able to tolerate physical discomfort, and approval seeking (Thompson & Sherman, 1993).

Epling and Pierce (1991) have suggested that, rather than being a result of the drive for thinness, physical activity in and of itself can be associated with, cause, or exacerbate anorexia. They have termed this condition *activity anorexia,* which they define as:

> the loss of appetite that occurs when physical activity interferes with eating. . . . The first effect of combining dieting and exercise is that physical activity accelerates to excessive levels. As exercise increases, the value of food declines and people eat less. Paradoxically, as food intake decreases (i.e., deprivation) the motivation to exercise increases. (Epling & Pierce, 1991, p. 111)

In a paradoxical manner, they suggested, food restriction increases physical activity; the activity affects physiological processes, and these in turn lead to increased food restriction. "Once initiated, this cycle of increasing activity and decreasing food intake is resistant to change" (Epling & Pierce, 1991, p. 9).

Epling and Pierce proposed that there may be physiological bases for this behavior. In evolutionary terms, activity as a response to starvation may have the functional value of increasing the likelihood of finding food. Endogenous opiates, potentially produced by exercise, may decrease appetite. Because of cultural conditioning, women more than men are likely to use diet and exercise in such a way that the biobehavioral process of activity anorexia is initiated. "Activity anorexia is therefore a biobehavioral process activated by cultural requirements for thinness and fitness" (Epling & Pierce, 1991, p. 168).

PRACTITIONER RECOMMENDATIONS

As with bulimic clients, when exercise takes on a different function, and even becomes symptomatic, it is important to help clients discontinue its destructive use and subsequently to assist clients in moving toward healthy, or at least moderated, exercise. A number of inpatient programs prohibit exercise among anorexic patients, but enforcement may be challenging. This prohibition can serve merely as an alternate arena for the same type of power struggles as occur around food intake. Beumont, Beumont, Touyz, and Williams suggested that a supervised exercise program for anorexic and bulimic patients can serve "the major goal of therapy—namely, to facilitate the patients' responsibility for themselves, rather than to increase feelings of helplessness, resentment, and dependence" (1997, p. 186).

Physical activity that is viewed as part of the reconnection between self and body can serve a therapeutic function. To the extent that there are physiological or compulsive aspects of exercise for the anorexic client, yoga or walking may be especially helpful. These forms of exercise may involve less energy expenditure and can enhance attention to one's self in the present moment.

Disordered Eating Patterns and Mixed Diagnoses

A short, stocky 19-year-old, Tammy lost 60 pounds rapidly through severe food restriction. Two years later, she entered group and then individual therapy with marked depression, severe fatigue, and health complications from her underweight and chronic underfed condition. She severely restricted eating, with an intermixed pattern of 3 days of fasting followed by brief episodes of voracious, although limited, eating with subsequent purging by vomiting.

Following a successful hospitalization on an eating disorders unit, she continued somewhat restrictive with regard to eating. However, she began making active strides around age-appropriate separation from her dysfunctional family of origin. She became increasingly assertive at work and in relationships. Many of her unfolding plans and intentions needed to be reassessed, however, when she found out, to her dismay, that she was pregnant.

Needing to put many of her newfound skills into play in unanticipated ways, Tammy returned to her parents' home, at the same time setting more appropriate interpersonal boundaries with them and her boyfriend. She began walking regularly, along with other aspects of improved self-care, including reasonable eating. We framed the self-care in terms of "feeding" herself— physically, emotionally, and mentally. Toward the latter stage of pregnancy, she experienced increased joint pain and found that this was eased by walking.

As she began dealing postpartum with the residual weight effects of pregnancy, Tammy struggled between her two models of weight management: her earlier, ineffective but seemingly successful method of not eating and her more recent attention to hunger signals and balanced eating. She knew from past experience that enervation was one of the net effects of severe food restriction. She recognized that she needed to maintain energy in order to cope with child care, work, and new definitions of relationships. She compromised on one meal a day, and alleviated her anxiety about having eaten, often, by going for a 4-mile walk, at her mother's urging, and often accompanied by her mother. She was aware that she felt better both physically and psychologically.

Tammy's case illustrates a number of aspects common among the general population of women with eating issues. Although anorexia nervosa and bulimia nervosa are diagnostically separate entities, the distinction between these two disorders is in actuality often arbitrary (Walsh & Garner, 1997). In my outpatient practice, I find that many of the eating disordered women with whom I work have developed over time a conglomerate of disordered eating patterns and food and weight preoccupation. Three or 10 or 20 years of disregulated eating creates and reinforces a blend of food preoccupation, distorted body perception, shame, passivity, and low self-esteem that is simultaneously predictable and idiosyncratic. These characteristics are inextricably entwined with various ineffective and self-maintaining systems of starvation, overeating, and purging.

As with Tammy and Diana, whether causally linked or associated, comorbid psychiatric conditions may be present as well. Depression is perhaps most frequent, along with anxiety disorders, particularly obsessive-compulsive disorder (Crowther & Sherwood, 1997). Familial, if not personal, engagement with substance abuse, and a history of childhood sexual abuse or other trauma, often seem present as well (Fallon & Wonderlich, 1997; Mitchell, Specker, & Edmonson, 1997). There are complex chicken and egg issues regarding etiology, diagnosis, and treatment. Yet as I illustrate in other chapters in this section, exercise is often a useful aspect of treatment for any of these conditions.

The psychotherapy goal for eating disordered women who distort exercise should not be the elimination of exercise. Rather, changes in exercise patterns are a part of the change of focus on the self and the body. Moving toward an appreciation of herself as having value and worth in her own being, the client becomes able to attend to those aspects of her life that will help her feel healthy. Exercise is one such component. Instead of exercise as self-flagellation, the woman can begin to tap into the pleasure inherent in movement. At least initially, however, she will need to continue to guard against her old habits. She can make use of the seductive pull of overexercise as a cue to the ways in which her life may be feeling out of control. Symptom then becomes signal, allowing opportunity for change.

Pacing Oneself: 11
Exercise and Substance Abuse Recovery

T he pairing of substance abuse and exercise typically brings to mind the variety of ways in which athletes use and abuse substances. And the vast majority of literature regarding the interaction of substances and exercise focuses on the compromising effects of alcohol or other substances (e.g., steroids) on athletes, rather than the use of exercise in the process of recovery. Although I discuss some of those issues in chapter 17, here I focus on ways in which exercise can be used as people discontinue substance abuse.

Alcohol and Drug Abuse Recovery

Alcohol and drug problems are endemic. Approximately 10% of adults in the United States have significant problems with alcohol, and one quarter of American adults regularly use tobacco (Miller & Brown, 1997). Further, substance use disorders are comorbid with many other mental disorders such that up to one half of clients being treated for medical and psychological problems may have significant alcohol or other drug involvement. Likewise, alcohol- or other drug abuse-dependence is a major risk factor for other diagnosable mental health problems (Miller & Brown, 1997).

Although research information on effective psychological treatments is available, training biases and a moralistic tradition have left much of the treatment to popular but unsubstantiated methods. Yet many of the most effective alcohol or other substance abuse treatments focus on issues related to risk for relapse, including social skills training, relapse prevention, and stress management (Miller & Brown, 1997). Each of these treatments can incorporate the use of exercise as one component.

In one of the few experimental studies of the effect of aerobic exercise (or meditation) on alcohol consumption, Murphy, Pagano, and Marlatt (1986) randomly assigned 60 male college students who were heavy social drinkers to an 8-week treatment intervention: exercise (running), meditation, or a no-treatment control group. Although there was an attrition rate of 50% among all groups, participants in the running condition significantly reduced their alcohol consumption, especially during weekdays, equivalent to drinking 14 fewer drinks per week. This behavioral change was apparently related to opportunity for timeout, time to oneself, sense of accomplishment, and increased self-worth. Among those who were at a high level of compliance with meditation, this method was also effective. Even when they did not look forward to running or meditation, participants noted in their journals that they felt less tense and much more relaxed, had an increased sense of well-being, and slept better after running or meditation.

Decreased anxiety and depression, as well as higher rates of abstinence, have been noted following physical exercise programs in inpatient substance abuse treatment programs (Kremer, Malkin, & Benshoff, 1995). The authors suggested that since substance abuse behaviors often occur during leisure time, physical activity can provide healthy alternatives. In a survey of injection drug users enrolled in an HIV and AIDS prevention program, one participant commented that involvement in exercise or sports helps reduce stress and serves as a reciprocal inhibitor: "If you are involved in sports, you don't have time to be involved in drugs or around people involved in drugs" (Powers, Woody, & Sachs, 1999).

A daily exercise program, conducted for 6 weeks at an inpatient rehabilitation center for alcoholics, resulted at 3-month follow-up in a significantly higher abstinence rate (69% vs. 38% in comparable programs), improved capacity to cope with emotional stress, greater responsivity to the psychotherapy conducted during inpatient treatment, and subsequent reorganization of leisure time (Sinyor, Brown, Rostant, & Seraganian, 1982). Although this was not a controlled experiment, the powerful effects of exercise with this population appear impressive.

One of the earliest to focus on the positive interaction of exercise and substance use reduction, a psychiatrist, William Glasser (1976), popularized the idea that "positive addiction" could be used as a substitute for "negative addiction." Broadly defined, positive addiction helps strengthen people and facilitates increased life satisfaction. Negative addictions such as substance abuse, in contrast, weaken people and may destroy them. From anecdotal reports, he suggested that physical addictions, such as running, may be especially beneficial in discontinuing alcohol or smoking. In response to a questionnaire he developed, a businessman, formerly "an almost hopeless alcoholic" who had discontinued drinking now felt that running had completely destroyed any desire to drink. The man commented, in relation to running: "I am always energetic and enthusiastic. I think quicker and clearer. I always feel like I always wanted to feel by having a few drinks" (p. 120).

In a survey of more than 700 readers of *Running Times*, Johnsgard noted a significant decrease in concern about addictions—alcohol, drugs, or cigarettes—over time for both men and women. With the exception of one woman, "the men and women who had begun to run in order to kick alcohol or nicotine dependency made it" (1989, p. 47).

At a more personal level, George Sheehan spoke to the effect of running on his alcohol use:

> Distance running . . . was a positive factor and the decisive one. Negative injunctions never work. Lives are changed by do's, not don'ts. And if one is to stop drinking permanently, one must be actively involved in becoming what one is. Distance running did that for me. It reintroduced me to my body. And my body, I found out, had a mind of its own. It would no longer accept anything less than the best. . . . Having reached the peak of its powers, it dragged my mind and my will along with it. (1978, p. 49)

Some inpatient and outpatient programs are founded on such an assumption. The Adventure Network, near Philadelphia, for example, offers various combinations of adventure-based counseling and outdoor education, using the challenge and adventure inherent in group activities such as ropes courses, caving, rock climbing, and kayaking. One of its programs in particular, Adventures in Sobriety, is offered to individuals involved in Twelve Step programs, rehabilitation drug and alcohol rehabilitation centers, and high school and college groups. Therapeutic recreation professionals have created a national network, Therapeutic Recreators for Recovery, and provide both inpatient and oupatient therapeutic recreation programs, including walking, games, sports, weight training, and aerobics.

Because of running's addictive potential, Greist and colleagues (1979) suggested that running therapy could be an effective replacement therapy for various substance addictions. They reported two

I run because of the joy of running, the poetry of the sunrise. I run about 20 miles per week and bike from 100–200+ miles per week. If I had to choose between running and bicycling, I would not be able to do it.

I am a recovering alcoholic, in my 21st year of continuous sobriety. Drinking is no longer an option, like driving a car without a seat belt, biking without a helmet, or wearing poor shoes when running. One just doesn't do these things.

Running got me sober and has kept me sober—I don't think AA would have been sufficient. I began running in 1972, when my doctor told me to exercise or die. As my disease of alcoholism progressed, I began missing races, through the usual blackouts. Because I hated mssing races, in 1978 I got to AA. AA is great for the beginner but the #$%^ cigarette smoke and Lord's [sic] prayer were turn offs and I disengaged after I had survived that critical first year. Although many people in AA weren't enthusiastic about my running, I have continued running. It's my idea that the people who stay sober have some overriding passion in their lives like exercise.

61-year-old female psychologist

earlier studies of hospitalized alcoholics who showed considerable improvement in cardiovascular fitness and other physiological measures of fitness, self-esteem, and sleep over a 3-week period of daily jogging. In one of the groups, exercise may have been related as well to decreased length of hospitalization. Similarly, studies of exercise with severely disturbed hospitalized patients (Auchus, Wood, & Kaslow, 1995; Martinsen, Hoffart, & Solberg, 1989) described more completely in chapters 7 and 12, have included alcoholics among those patients.

In addition to being an aspect of recovery from substance abuse, exercise may be effective in preventing such problems. Danish, Nellen, and Owens (1996) pointed to an interactive cluster of health-compromising behaviors in adolescents, including drug and alcohol abuse, violent and delinquent behaviors, dangerous sexual practices, and school dropout. Yet potentially, primary prevention can disrupt this nascent cluster. By acquiring life skills associated with success, and learning health-enhancing behaviors, adolescents can learn what to say "yes" to (Danish, Nellen, & Owens, 1996, p. 208). Activity thus becomes a metaphor for enhancing competence.

A childhood and adolescence filled with interpersonal challenges and poor coping skills became the shaky foundation for Brian's troubling adulthood:

36-year-old Brian sought therapy concerning an intense grief reaction he experienced while breaking up with the woman he had been dating for the last 8 months. He felt that his response was disproportionate to the meaning of the relationship. "I don't need to be this devastated over this woman."

Intense and competitive, he had begun drinking and smoking marijuana in junior high school, had had an affair with one of his teachers in high school—and proudly announced that he was the first student ever expelled from his high school. He described his father as an active alcoholic, "but my mother keeps him under a tight rein." His father responded to Brian's expulsion by beating him severely. Brian left home, joined the Army, returned home, completed college, and joined the family business—all while continuing to drink heavily and use a variety of drugs.

Following a serious car accident at age 31, strung out on cocaine as well as alcohol, and still smoking heavily, Brian agreed to hospitalization for detoxification. He had been able to remain sober since that hospitalization, 5 years previously, and had also discontinued cigarettes 2 years previously.

Brian had become actively engaged in Alcoholics Anonymous (AA) at the time of hospitalization, and had maintained that association over this period of time. He also began riding his bicycle, and became involved with a local bicycle recreational riding and racing group.

It is interesting to speculate whether Brian's abstinence may be exercise-related in five separate but interacting ways:

1. Physiological: There continues to be considerable controversy about the function of endogenous opiods in affecting mood in relation to exercise, yet this possibility is one well worth considering. Hoffman (1997) suggested that "a program of physical activity, together with other interventions, might facilitate the conversion of the addict from dependence on alcohol or exogenous opiates to an 'endogenous endorphinist'" (p. 173).
2. Distraction: Drinking and using substances takes time. If one fills one's time with other activities (such as exercise), it can help one over the hump of down time.
3. Sociability: As with AA, Brian clearly cherished the peer friendships he developed in the biking club.
4. Focus and outlet for emotions: A chronically tense, aggressive, and competitive person, working out hard was a means of channeling a variety of his energies.
5. Mastery: Having chronically perceived himself as unworthy and inadequate, Brian relished the increased sense of competence he experienced through his sport activity.

As Brian continued to attempt to remain disengaged from his earlier relationship, his former girlfriend more actively pursued him. Concerned that he would succumb and restart the relationship, and uncomfortable about her continued heavy drinking, he felt anxious and agitated. Cautiously, he acquiesced to instruction in deep breathing. He was especially responsive to triangle breathing, and reported feeling an increased sense of relaxation. However, he was somewhat reluctant to use it outside of the office, saying that he liked to be in "high gear." A few weeks later, almost sheepishly, he commented that he had found the deep breathing helpful especially when he was feeling overstressed.

In preparation for a 100 mile road race a few months into treatment, Brian recalled having broken his collarbone at the 60 mile mark during this race the prior year. A generally superstitious person, he was sure that he would "bonk" at the same point this year as well. Often resistant to therapeutic suggestions, he was responsive to recommendations regarding the mental aspects of his training. He felt empowered by understanding the difference between associative and dissociative thinking. I also emphasized the immense changes he had been able to make in his own life. We spoke of the ways in which the persistence needed in maintaining sobriety could sustain him during the long bike race. The following week, Brian commented that he felt good about all 106 (!) of the miles he had ridden. In particular, he felt that he had paced himself well.

After the initial 4 months of fairly intense treatment, Brian had resolved his feelings about his dating partner, recognizing that he could not force his will of wishing her sober either on her or on their relationship. He thought that the most important message I had given him was to "lighten up." He continued, however, to be and see himself as highly competitive, needing to win in relationships as well as everyday life.

Brian contacted me for some brief treatment a number of times over the subsequent 4 years concerning various disastrous enmeshments and entanglements with women. Having approached and then passed his 40th birthday, he felt both more desperate and more resigned about not yet being married. He began dating a pleasant but not "high-maintenance" woman, a totally new experience for him. He continued to abstain from alcohol, drugs, and cigarettes. He was a regular "sponsor" within AA. Although still bike riding, he had now also become an avid racquetball player and saw the racquetball club as the source for many of his friendships.

The central focus of Brian's psychotherapy concerned relationship issues. At the same time, exercise was relevant to this psychotherapy. Support for his involvement with exercise, the application of various psychological skills methods in regard to anxiety management and competition, and exercise metaphor, all enriched therapy.

Smoking Cessation and Exercise

I had worked with 58-year-old Bonnie on a variety of issues over a long period of time, including marital distress and the management of a traumatic loss, when she came in for a "booster" session the day before a marker event related to the trauma. We discussed various strategies for handling this event. As the session proceeded, we also discussed her resumption of cigarette smoking. She described herself as finding smoking a waste of time. She was frustrated with herself for having resumed this habit at the time of trauma. Likewise, although she had at one point exercised regularly, she had not been exercising recently. Rather, in the morning she would find herself with a cup of coffee and 2 cigarettes, watching the morning news instead of using her exercise equipment. I suggested that she begin the morning by getting up and heading toward the equipment before her cup of coffee. Further, I suggested she start tomorrow morning. Which, I asked, would be better preparation for this difficult day: exercise or cigarettes?

Although she agreed with this assessment, there were not enough supports at that moment for Bonnie to make this behavioral shift. The situational stressors were so intense that, with the lack of others to support this behavioral shift, the word of her psychotherapist was not enough to impel change at that point.

Bonnie was still in the preparation stage of change, yet the fact that she had raised this issue around this significant event suggested that she was nearly ready to resume her prior exercise behavior and discontinue smoking. A month later, she eased back into regular morning exercise and tapered her smoking.

DISCUSSION

If there is little available information about the relationship between exercise and alcohol abstinence, there is even less with regard to exercise and smoking cessation. In a few pilot studies, Marcus and colleagues (e.g., Marcus et al., 1995) noted that community-recruited women smokers who engaged in a 12-week exercise program were significantly more likely to quit than a contact control group (40% vs. 5%). Likewise, they were significantly more likely to continue abstinent 12 months later (25% vs. 5%). In some instances, as with Bonnie, above, exercise and cigarette smoking may compete for time and as a method of mood control. At other times, the relationship may be antithetical. Exercise may lead to a decreased interest in smoking, or, more typically, people who discontinue smoking may start exercising. Occasionally, there is a flash of inspired substitution of one habit for the other:

> Running to catch a bus, almost missing it, and severely out of breath, Jonathan wondered if he was having a heart attack. As his heartbeat slowed and he regained his composure, he flung away his cigarettes, vowed he would stop smoking, and embarked on running on a daily basis. Twelve years and 10 marathons later, he has continued not to smoke and finds it hard to remember his former self.

After an adolescent hiatus, a woman friend challenged me to run 1 mile in college. As a smoker and an overweight athlete, but still one of those adolescents with an immortality complex, I took the challenge, ran the mile, collapsed at the end, and realized the sad shape of things. . . . I actually liked the feeling of running and took it up regularly. A short while later, I experienced a personal trauma; running and swimming became my personal ways to feel control and power over my life, my self. So I ran with it.

44-year-old female psychologist

The synergistic potential for various health behaviors programmatically designed for adolescents (Danish, Nellen, & Owens, 1996) can manifest in adults as well. For example, in extolling the natural body rhythms of exercise, Sheehan (1978) commented: "The athlete doesn't stop smoking and start training. He starts training and finds he has stopped smoking. The athlete doesn't go on a diet and start training. He starts training and finds he is eating the right things at the right time" (p. 56). In a random survey of marathoners who had previously smoked, 81% of the men and 75% of the women stopped smoking when they began running. For men, there was a correlation between probability of smoking cessation and weekly mileage (Crandall, 1986). Reflecting on one of the respondents in his survey, a man who had quit a 2–3 pack per day habit 4 months into running, Glasser suggested that running was as incompatible with smoking as it was with worrying. More typically, however, people may quit smoking because it interferes with their lung capacity and endurance once they have started exercise.

There are a number of reasons why beginning to exercise as one discontinues smoking may be especially beneficial (Garland DeNelsky, personal communication, March 11, 1998):

- Exercise aids weight control, both through direct burning of calories and the metabolic shift that can occur.
- Exercise serves as an excellent barometer that provides feedback as to how one's body is recovering from the effects of smoking.
- Exercise can provide some of the mood-enhancing effects previously obtained from nicotine.

PRACTITIONER RECOMMENDATIONS

Although there is little empirical research on the use of exercise with regard to the discontinuation of substance abuse, anecdote and logic suggest a synergistic relationship between substance discontinuation and exercise. As indicated above, the recommendation of exercise potentially may serve a number of functions, including distraction, attention to health and recovery, positive biochemical effects, mastery and persistence, the management of social isolation, and mood regulation.

For those who have become physically debilitated from years of drinking or drug ingestion as well as a lifestyle involving little exercise and poor nutrition, Kremer and colleagues (1995) suggested that walking may be an especially appropriate form of exercise. It is not physically stressful. Further, walking can easily be suited to a group activity, thus enhancing social skill development.

Because health functioning, including heart, lungs, or liver, may be compromised as a result of substance abuse, a thorough physical examination prior to engaging in exercise is essential.

"Burning Off Negative Thoughts":
Exercise for People With Chronic Mental Illness

12

A pproximately 5.4 million people in the United States (just below 3% of the adult population) have a severe and persistent mental illness (National Advisory Mental Health Council, 1990). People with chronic and severe mental illness tend to have high rates of physical illness; poor general or cardiovascular fitness; obesity; and sluggishness, low energy, poor body image, and low self-concept (Pelham & Campagna, 1991; Unger, Skrinar, Hutchinson, & Yelmokas, 1992).

> The main leisure activities of an individual who has been ill with a schizophrenic disorder are watching television, writing, reading, or listening to music. These activities may be enjoyable and creative, but are sedentary and solitary with little vocational application. They reinforce the secondary dysfunctions associated with schizophrenia, such as social withdrawal and seclusiveness. (Pelham & Campagna, 1991, p. 167)

Physical activity has beneficial impact with regard to the syndromic features of mental illness, even if it does not affect the illness itself. Thus, if only in regard to the secondary or associated effects, the use of exercise with this population would seem potentially of value.

A negative correlation between mental illness and physical fitness has long been noted. In one of the earliest studies in exercise psychology, in 1934 Linton, Hamelink, and Hoskins (reported in Rejeski & Thompson, 1993) found the cardiovascular fitness of a group of hospitalized patients with schizophrenia to be significantly poorer than that of a control group of hospital staff. They attributed this difference to the inactivity of hospitalized patients. More recently, Unger and colleagues (Unger et al., 1992) suggested that both inactivity and social isolation may be a function of any number of additional factors, including the psychomotor retardation that may be symptomatic of severe depression, diet deficiencies, or the effect of certain psychotropic medications. A study of 15 patients in a multidisciplinary psychiatric rehabilitation program (Pelham, Campagna, Ritvo, & Birnie, 1993) noted a significant negative correlation between predicted aerobic fitness and level of depression (Beck Depression Inventory [BDI]), indicating that higher levels of aerobic fitness corresponded to lower levels of depression.

> Marcia, a 24-year-old single woman, started taking lithium following her first manic episode. Soon after, she began gaining weight and discontinued her medication without telling her psychiatrist. Within 2 months, she had been rehospitalized, suffering from another manic episode.
>
> After she was stabilized, the psychiatrist and social worker reviewed with her the precipitants to the second episode. Marcia admitted that she had stopped taking the lithium because of weight gain while on the medication. The social worker, who had herself struggled to maintain a healthy weight, suggested that daily exercise could counteract the weight gain caused by the lithium.
>
> While still in the hospital, Marcia began a supervised aerobic and weight training regimen. She made plans to join a local gym upon discharge. The daily exercise did not completely counter the weight-stimulating effects of the lithium. However, it minimized the impact to the extent that Marcia was willing to continue with both. Now, 3 years later, she is still on lithium, works out daily, and has not experienced a subsequent manic episode.

The subject of exercise for people with severe and chronic mental illness has received astoundingly little attention in the psychotherapeutic literature. Those studies that exist tend to be descriptive pilot studies, with small numbers and few if any controls (Auchus & Kaslow, 1994; Auchus, Wood, & Kaslow, 1995; Pelham & Campagna,1991; Unger et al., 1992). As with exercise in relation to substance abuse users, exercise for people with severe or chronic mental illness appears to be handled primarily as therapeutic recreation, rather than as an aspect of the psychotherapeutic armamentarium.

Yet it is striking that even the most distressed among us experience exercise as salubrious, affecting mood, mind, and body. Indigent psychiatric inpatients gave the following comments about exercise: "Like I had more energy to do what I had to do, when I don't walk I feel real sluggish." "More energized." "Makes me burn off negative thoughts." "Clears my thinking." "Always seems to make you feel better" (Auchus, Wood, & Kaslow, 1995, p. 139).

Although criteria and definitions vary, in this chapter I consider research reports of those with severe psychiatric disabilities including people with chronic schizophrenia, as well as mood, substance abuse, and personality disorders. The latter three diagnoses do not in and of themselves imply severe or chronic mental illness. However, the participants in the studies reported here with these diagnoses either experienced severe forms of these disorders or had undergone psychiatric hospitalization, or both. Information concerning patients with milder forms of mood disorder is located in chapter 7.

In a detailed case description, Mirella Auchus (1993) serendipitously noted the psychotherapeutic effects that occurred among members of a weight lifting group for seriously disturbed psychiatric outpatients. She suggested that a weight lifting group may be effective in part because the structured and tangible nature of weight lifting means that goal and task identification are readily apparent. Bonding and trust occur with both the leader and other group members through requisite shared activities such as spotting. The therapist-weight trainer functions, additionally, as a catalyst for increasing members' confidence and self-esteem, as well as providing education and reality testing, all functions of a group therapist. Further, natural role modeling occurs, as well as the literal and metaphoric function of a holding environment. "The weight lifting group created an environment that nurtured and enhanced members' abilities and did not focus on disabilities" (p. 31).

Among the effects Auchus noted were:

1. Social role transformation, in which participants' sense of identity could expand beyond the self-limiting one of patient or nonperson within society to include weight lifter as well;
2. Interpersonal interaction, shifting from an initial position of parallel play to a shared common project of improved muscular strength and endurance;
3. An opportunity to play and be playful in a way that was experienced as meaningful;
4. Enhanced structure and discipline through adherence to the structure and sequencing of the weight lifting sessions;
5. Increased responsibility, initiative, group problem solving, teamwork, and camaraderie, interpersonal commitment, and a sense of belonging. "Individuals who suffer from serious psychiatric disabilities often do not have a place where they 'fit in'" (1993, p. 35);

6. Increased interest in health related issues, such as nutrition and healthy eating.

Coming to some of these same conclusions, Pelham and Campagna (1991) described three patients with chronic schizophrenia seen at a psychiatric rehabilitation clinic. Exercise was designed to enhance fitness, weight, and energy, and provide drug alternatives. As well, exercise may serve to counteract the social, as well as psychological, isolation endemic to such patients. Initially, each of Pelham and Campagna's patients worked on exercise on a one-to-one basis with an exercise therapist. The goal was eventual transfer to a homogeneous group and then heterogeneous groups within the general population. To increase the likelihood of social interaction and identification with the general (nonchronic schizophrenic) public, the patients were encouraged to swim during open swim times, or participate in pick-up games. Aware of available community organizations and activities, the exercise therapist helped match each patient to appropriate community resources. All three patients ultimately engaged in a variety of activities in public settings.

In identifying patients likely to respond to the program, Pelham and Campagna found that key factors were personal past experience with exercise or sport as well as a positive attitude about the benefits of exercise. Martinsen (1990) also noted the positive effect of previous adult experience with exercise as predictive of long-term therapeutic response to exercise among hospitalized patients.

After 8 weeks of exercise 4 times a week, eleven patients in a rehabilitation program with diagnoses of schizophrenia or major affective disorder indicated in interview that they were experiencing anxiolytic, antidepressant, and energizing effects (Pelham et al., 1993). Patients also observed that exercise helped them become more motivated in regard to other components of their rehabilitation program. Although almost all patients reported positive responses to the exercise program, those engaged in aerobic exercise (cycle ergometer) were significantly more enthusiastic than those engaged in muscle tone and strengthening exercises. In a subsequent study that compared the effects among 10 patients randomly assigned to aerobic or nonaerobic exercise for 12 weeks, those in the aerobic program dramatically improved aerobic fitness (probably because of initial below average fitness). Additionally, there were significant reductions in BDI scores. The group engaging in nonaerobic exercise neither increased their aerobic fitness nor reduced their BDI scores.

Young adult undergraduate students (mean age 33) with psychiatric disabilities and an average of 17 months of prior hospitalization had the opportunity to enroll in a 10-week supervised fitness training

> Approximately 5 out of 20 patients who I work with at the state hospital faithfully do minor exercises five times a week. Approximately 2 out of 14 will participate in an individually designed exercise program.
>
> I haven't found any disadvantages to exercising with the patients, although I know some staff who exercise with mental patients feel embarrassed for their own shortcomings. Embarrassing things happen—bra straps fall down, stomachs show, men's underwear show, etc.
>
> **57-year-old female psychologist**

program designed to measure the effect of fitness training on cardiovascular fitness, body fat, and self-esteem (Skrinar, Unger, Hutchinson, & Faigenbaum, 1992; Unger et al., 1992). Of 40 potential participants, 9 volunteered and, ultimately, 6 completed the program. Students participated in the program twice a week, and "compliance to the program was exemplary" (Unger et al., 1992, p. 24). Cardiovascular fitness improved significantly, body composition showed some improvement, and, although the self-report questionnaire did not reflect change in self-esteem, "participants described positive attitudinal and behavior changes not reported by the assessment tool" (p. 25). During an exit interview, all students described themselves as feeling much better, and "statements were made about improved mental status, decreased anxiety, improved coping, increased self-esteem, and increased energy level" (p. 25), in addition to the pleasure derived from socialization through group participation.

Although the students decreased their exercise frequency 4 months after the program ended, all students reportedly were interested in resuming regular exercise. Nutritional changes and the ability to handle stress had been maintained. A year later, two of the students had enrolled in a fitness program and all described some level of physical activity. Having reverted to the contemplation or preparation stages of change, with some minor supports, the students were excellent candidates for developing lifestyle change. Although this was clearly a very limited sample from the potential pool, it adds support to the idea that self-selected exercise programs can have a powerful impact on people with psychiatric disabilities.

Exercise and Medication

There are a number of issues with regard to the relationship between exercise and psychotropic medication among the chronically and severely mentally ill. There are concerns about adapting exercise to the needs of those on medication, as well as the potential for exercise to supplement if not supplant medication.

Skrinar et al. (1992) pointed to the challenge of maintaining exercise while taking one or more psychotropic medications. In their study, these medications included Artane, Ativan, Elavil, Haldol, Lithium, Lithium Carbonate, Loxitane, Prolixin, and Xanax. Potential side effects of these medications that could interfere with functional exercise include, among others, muscular rigidity, dehydration, muscle weakness, fatigue, and impaired coordination. Since medications such as tricyclic antidepressants can have cardiovascular side effects, exercise programs have tended to screen for pre-existing cardiovascular disease, moderate the intensity of exercise, and continue monitoring cardiovascular side effects during the program (Martinsen, 1990; Pelham & Campagna, 1991).

What of the possibility that exercise may become an alternative to the use of medication among such patients? Since long-term use of many of the more potent psychotropic medications may result in serious but potentially reversible side effects, drug "holidays" are sometimes recommended. During those times, Pelham and Campagna (1991) suggested that a program of aerobic exercise could be especially effective in retaining some of the effects normally derived from medication. Pelham and colleagues (1993) further commented: "Several clients responded favorably to exercise in association with withdrawal of medication, supporting the notion that exercise may have a salient, independent therapeutic effect in some clients. For example, the three clients who were able to withdraw from phenothiazine medication remained medication free for the duration of the studies" (p. 81).

Caution needs to be taken regarding these findings, as the numbers of patients, types of illness, and types and dosages of medication have not been systematically studied. There is still considerable research to be done on exercise mode, specific psychopathology, dose-response relationship of exercise to psychiatric disability, and type and dosage of medication (Skrinar et al., 1992)

Patients' Perspective

In each of the studies described here, the self-report experience of the vast majority of patients who exercise tends to be positive. For example, after hospital discharge, a person with schizophrenia remarked: "When you do a workout it gives you drive, makes you work harder, your drive is stronger. It makes you want to do other things. More you do, the more you can do. It makes you feel good, feel great. . . . If you are worrying about something you ride it out" (Pelham & Campagna, 1991, p. 163). Of 50 low-income patients hospitalized at a crisis stabilization unit, 41 (82%) reported that they exercised, primarily walking, one to five times a week at a moderate level of intensity (Auchus, Wood, & Kaslow, 1995). Of the 41, 78% indicated that they felt better following exercise. The unusually high number of patients who reported exercising were probably combining intentional exercise with walking as a modality for transportation (Auchus, personal communication, April 17, 1998). Similarly, day program participants who were engaged in a weight lifting group all reported improved mood ("better" or "much better" on a 5-point Likert type scale) as well as showing significant improvement in muscular strength and endurance (Auchus & Kaslow, 1994). Scores on the Zung Self-Rating Depression Scale remained in the nondepressed range, suggesting that there was no exacerbation of psychiatric symptoms during the program.

Practitioner Recommendations

Although the literature on the use of exercise with people with severe and chronic mental illness is limited, it is important to note that in none of the reports is there concern about the exacerbation of mental illness through or in response to exercise. It appears that, with appropriate recognition of the increased need for medical monitoring, exercise for this population is both safe and effective. Regarding the use of exercise as an alternative to medication, at this time there appears to be insufficient research evidence on the subject for the nonmedical mental health practitioner to make such a recommendation. However, if such a program is undertaken, the psychotherapist may be in an excellent position to evaluate patients' behavioral responses.

The psychologist in such a setting may be in the role of assisting in the design of such a program, as compared with carrying it out directly. In this regard, it is especially important to engage the involvement of a multidisciplinary team that includes exercise physiologists, leisure or recreation counselors, and health care personnel.

Certain characteristics seem to make such programs most effective. A program of graduated training recognizes the likelihood that initially participants may be physically deconditioned. Social interaction serves an important program function. There is mixed evidence concerning the effectiveness on mental well-being of aerobic as compared with anaerobic exercise. In designing a program, individual preference may well be a key factor in determining effectiveness.

Idiosyncratic responses and attributions may occur among program participants. The college students, for example, apparently experienced undue initial anxiety about the laboratory equipment and exercise testing protocols (Skrinar et al., 1992). Thus, gradual introduction to community or private facilities and full explanation of equipment and facilities may be an important component of any program that is begun with this population.

From Being Alive to Feeling Alive: Trauma Survivor Empowerment

13

To the extent that exercise and psychotherapy seem like an unanticipated match, exercise for trauma survivors may appear to be an even more unlikely combination. People who are dealing with the sequelae of recent or distant traumatic issues tend to be caught in various entangling mental processes, perhaps to a greater extent than among other therapy populations. The body may seem irrelevant to the process of therapy. Further, when one's body has been the site of betrayal, clients may feel especially disinclined to focus on the body and its functioning. The Aristotelian dichotomy between mind and body may be exacerbated through dissociative processes that often are endemic to the trauma experience (Freyd, 1996; Herman, 1992; Pope & Brown, 1996). Additionally, performance enhancement training, designed to improve already good skills for future performance, would seem to contrast with trauma work that has a rehabilitative focus.

And yet, both exercise and sport psychology can be of considerable value to the practitioner working with trauma survivors. Exercise may directly positively affect some of the psychological effects of trauma. Exercise, additionally, can mediate some

> Basically, if a person is inactive, I encourage him or her to look at the definition of self and how the physical aspect fits into that. I always recommend that a person consult with a physician about baseline health issues to get recommendations or possible restrictions concerning exercise.
>
> **44-year-old female psychologist**

of the associated conditions of trauma (e.g., depression, anxiety, low self-esteem). Furthermore, some of the techniques of psychological skills training can be of both general and specific use with this population.

In this chapter I address trauma survivor empowerment in two ways. I describe the use of exercise with trauma survivors first. Second, I discuss ways in which specific psychological skills methods typically used in sport psychology can be used with trauma survivors. I consider issues with regard to athletes and sexual abuse, another layer of connection, in chapter 17.

Exercise and Trauma Recovery

It has been suggested that people function with three central core beliefs or schemas: the world is seen as, and anticipated to continue being, essentially (a) benevolent and (b) meaningful, and (c) the self has worth (Janoff-Bulman, 1992). Trauma is characterized by disruption (rather than a gradual change over time) of a person's fundamental assumptions about the world. Stability and predictability are disrupted. The world becomes understood to be maleficent and meaningless, in which the self is abased. The net psychological effect of trauma is the shattering of the three core beliefs. The ultimate task of therapy for trauma involves the reconstruction of "a coherent system of meaning and belief that encompasses the story of the trauma" (Herman, 1992, p. 213).

Coping and recovery from trauma can be enhanced by increasing one's ability to tolerate arousal and distressing emotions; reworking and integrating information into one's sense of the world; and receiving the support of caring others (Janoff-Bulman, 1992). In the process of recovery, exercise may be helpful at both primary and secondary levels.

Exercise can help regulate physiological arousal, provide distraction from symptoms, and support a new sense of connection with the body. This development of caring connection with oneself can be benevolently described as "narcissistic attachment" (Weiss, 1975). Further, exercise may alleviate anxiety and depression. These diagnostic categories tend to co-act with posttraumatic stress disorder (PTSD). Exercise often has positive impact with regard to self-esteem, mastery, and body image, each of which may be compromised because of trauma.

An exploration of the potential utility of exercise for Vietnam war veterans with PTSD suggested that exercise might be effective in reducing social isolation, modulating high intensity affect, and reduc-

> When I exercise I find that my mind gets clear of much of its clutter, allowing me to focus on issues and ideas. The pace gets slowed down. I do not have the need to solve anything, just to sit with it. In doing so I typically have very clear and powerful insights about problems, solutions, and new ideas. It feels like cognitive clarity!
>
> There is a qualitative aspect to this process. I feel like I get in touch with my whole being—with the world. I leave logic and analytical thinking behind. I sit with the process of life, which to me is more qualitative in nature.
>
> **41-year-old female psychologist**

ing depression (Butcher, 1993). In a quasi-experimental study of 17 female therapy clients who were survivors of sexual abuse (Guerin, 1993), one half engaged in various forms of exercise, and one half did not. Although standardized personality and symptom measures did not indicate change, a number of qualitative effects were reported among the exercisers, including generally positive feelings about exercise; improved self-care (decreased alcohol and drug use, decreased binge eating, improved sleep); use of intentional dissociative techniques during exercise; and increased physical strength.

Adventure challenge programs have been developed specifically for trauma survivors. Some years ago, for example, I joined with two instructors in rock climbing to guide six participants in an Incest Survivors' Rock Climbing weekend (Hays, 1991). The two rock faces that were climbed were given, for the day, symbolic names: "Just Trust" and "Empowerment." The metaphor in action included encouragement from one of the instructors: "You can't see where you're going until you take the next step." "By the end of the day everyone's body feels stretched to the limits of its endurance. Emotionally, everyone is exceptionally serene and tranquil. Each woman has learned many lessons about her strengths and her vulnerabilities as well. The community of women is strengthened" (p. 15).

Because a number of issues may be involved, the inclusion of an exercise focus in treating individuals with an abuse history can be a complex undertaking. For treatment to be most effective, the therapist needs to carefully monitor meanings and attributions:

> With long loose hair and wildly painted fingernails, like a slightly older sister to the high school students she taught, 26-year-old Kris sought treatment initially around food and weight preoccupation. During the first few sessions, she detailed a family history lacking in nurturance, protection, or social and emotional skills education. In the context of this developmental bewilderment, she experienced two instances of sexual abuse, one by her father and one by a revered authority figure. Neither situation was acknowledged or dealt with at the time. Kris felt fragile, vulnerable, gullible, and naive. Maintaining this emotional immaturity, she felt, "I don't have the tools to nurture myself." Further, she connected this sense of herself as

unprotected to her weight. "I have felt that every man in my life is dangerous," she commented, "especially if I weigh less than 140 pounds. I'm not acknowledging the power I have as an adult woman to be safe. And yet I'd like to feel affirmed in the skills of an adult woman. I'd like to work through the issues of my body, really feel it, and as a result be thinner and have the body that works best for me."

Kris was bright, eager to change, and fairly transparent to herself in her defenses. Perhaps in part because she had done considerable trauma therapy during college, she was able to move from a detailed, cathartic telling of the specific incidents of sexual betrayal to focus on methods of self-soothing other than food. One obvious candidate was exercise. Through physical activity, she could redirect focus on the body toward its positive functioning and support her desire to let weight loss emerge as she felt more capable.

Kris had already begun walking regularly, and I supported this. She was feeling scared, however, that as she walked and started to lose weight, she was becoming "smaller." To her this implied disempowerment. What other image could she use to experience "smaller" or "slighter" as empowering, I asked? She thought that a sense of herself as becoming more like a sleek cat, perhaps a leopard, could work.

She tried this image out, and reported the following week that the image of a tiger seemed more apt. She found herself saying this "tiger"ness to herself, feeling silent but purring with it. The strength and power of this image allowed—in fact supported—her maintenance of walking. She could become thinner and stronger, physically and emotionally.

Psychological Skills Training With Trauma Survivors

A number of cognitive-behavioral methods and techniques are standard components of mental skills training programs with athletes. (Many of the terms used in this section are defined in the Glossary.) To illustrate the utility of these techniques with clinical populations, I describe a variety of them here with reference to resolution of trauma.

AROUSAL MANAGEMENT AND SELF-REGULATION THROUGH BREATHING AND RELAXATION TECHNIQUES

Arousal management, the keystone of effective performance, is likewise critical to the effective conduct of therapy with trauma survivors.

The same general principles apply to psychotherapy clients as to athletes: The classic inverted-U suggests that optimal performance will occur at a middle level of arousal; Hanin's concept of a "zone of optimal functioning" further refines this general principle to suggest that there are individual differences in preferred levels of arousal for specific tasks (Taylor, 1996). In regard to therapy, if a client is overly anxious, defensive maneuvers may block therapeutic progress. If a client is, alternatively, minimally engaged and experiencing no tension with regard to the presenting issues, there is little energy for the work of therapy.

Psychotherapy, then, functions best when the client is focused yet not flooded with anxiety. The regulation of levels of hyperarousal, a frequent component of PTSD, is of critical importance not only to the actual process of treatment for trauma survivors, but also to the client's functioning in everyday life. Training in deep breathing and other relaxation techniques can create an internal atmosphere of trust and safety, as well as personal control and empowerment (McCann & Pearlman, 1990).

ATTENTIONAL FOCUS AND CONCENTRATION

Problems in maintaining concentration, a major concern in sport performance, are often encountered by trauma survivors. In the "dialectic of trauma" (Herman, 1992), those with posttraumatic stress disorder may oscillate between intrusions of memory or affect and constriction, numbing, or detached consciousness. Dissociation, additionally, is a distressingly common experience. Techniques frequently used in sport settings can help ground a person in the present.

> Gloria, a 26-year-old with whom I had previously worked regarding a long history of physical, verbal, and sexual abuse by her alcoholic father, returned to therapy after having been raped by an acquaintance. She found herself easily panicked, distracted, and reactive. Although she had been free of dissociative symptoms for some time, in the face of this evocative stressor she felt tempted, as she described it, to "go over" into an alter personality. She was able to use the "pep cheer" to regain and maintain focus. The phrase "Where am I now? Here; What time is it? Now" became shortened to a mantralike "Here. Now." that quickly served to reorient her. As she focused on her present surroundings and current life, she could quiet the panic welling inside her.

Another simple technique to help a person regain control is to encourage them to concentrate for 10 seconds when they become aware that they have lost focus.

Claudia practiced this method when she became aware of feeling "spacey." Since one can only concentrate effectively on one thing at a time, she also developed an important internal attitude: "Only one frustration at a time. All the others will just have to wait."

ASSOCIATIVE AND DISSOCIATIVE STRATEGIES

Research concerning runners' cognitive styles suggests that some use associative strategies, focused on their bodily sensations, and others tend to think dissociatively, focused on anything but what their bodies are doing (Sachs, 1984a). This varies in part by level of skill as well as sport. An elite runner may use each body cue to give information about pacing; while putting in the miles, a recreational runner may solve work-related problems or mentally hum some music.

The clinical meaning of dissociation is, of course, somewhat different, referring to "an alteration of consciousness in which experiences and affects are not integrated into memory and awareness" (McCann & Pearlman, 1990, p. 41). Despite the semantic inconsistency of these terms, it is clear that treatment of trauma involves the management of phasic affective and cognitive functioning, which ranges between intrusion and constriction (Herman, 1992). The associative-dissociative strategies of sport psychology are thus akin to the handling of traumatic material through methods of approach and avoidance. There are benefits and costs to each: Approach allows increased assimilation of traumatic material but can become overwhelming; avoidance permits dosing of traumatic information but can be costly if the trauma remains unassimilated (McCann & Pearlman, 1990). Perhaps most important, clients come to learn that they have the capacity to regulate and develop voluntary control over the type and direction of their thought patterns, thus increasing their self-efficacy.

Jeanine, a 32-year-old woman in therapy for an extreme grief reaction following her mother's death, began experiencing intense outrage concerning a history of sibling incest and lack of parental protection. She found herself often filled with rage that, she understood intellectually, was unrelated to or out of proportion to a particular triggering incident. Although initially unable to modulate the intensity of that reaction, she found it helpful to understand that she had some choice about whether to stay emotionally engaged with the process or shift her focus at that particular moment. During cross-country skiing, she could focus on her heartbeat or stride (i.e., associate), or the quality of light and air (dissociate). With regard to her rage reactions, she could remain affectively embroiled, or shift her focus to other aspects of the current situation. To regain a sense of control of herself she began to consciously remove herself physically or emotionally from the situations in which she was overreacting. Later that day, she would cognitively explore the event that had triggered her reactions. Writing in her journal, she felt a much enhanced sense of self-control and self-understanding.

VISUALIZATION, GUIDED IMAGERY, AND MENTAL REHEARSAL

Visualization, perhaps the most popular depiction of sport psychology techniques, can be used for both mastery (imagining a perfect tennis match) or coping (behavioral rehearsal of the management of situations in which things go wrong) (Harris & Harris, 1984). These techniques, used judiciously, can be very powerful methods to rework trauma in a safe environment as well as practice new mental and behavioral skills (Courtois, 1988). (The use of imagery for the purpose of memory retrieval is at present considered quite controversial and is not advocated here [Enns et al., 1998; Pope & Brown, 1996]).

> I generally don't set aside time to visualize or self-coach as a dog exhibitor. When I am running, however, I often think about my dogs, and visualize a previous or upcoming competition with them, sort of "visualizing success." The rest of my life is very left hemisphere-dominated; exercise is when my right brain gets to kick in.
>
> **45-year-old male psychologist**

AFFIRMATIONS

Affirmations (e.g., "we're number one") are a regular part of psyching up. Short and specific, they seem to work best when they are individually developed, positive and realistic (or potentially so), have a rhythm or rhyme, and are framed in the present tense (Lynch, 1987).

> Forty-eight year-old Marcie was feeling extremely unfocused and tangential in her thinking. Anxiously avoidant, she often found herself overcome with a sensation of sleepiness. What's the opposite of sleepiness? I asked. "Energetic." We developed a phrase she could use: "I am energetic and focused." As she practiced this statement to herself, she found herself adding ". . . and I'm worth it."

TRANSITIONAL OBJECTS

The New York City Marathon Psyching Team consists of a group of volunteer psychotherapists who provide psychological skills training to the runners prior to this annual autumn event (Bloom, 1998; Runner's World, 1987). In order to keep track of marathoners using the

Psyching Team, Duane and Selman, the organizers, developed a method for easy identification and follow-up at the end of the race: Psyching Team members pin a piece of chute tape to runners' singlets at the conclusion of each brief intervention. The tape has taken on superstitious properties, such that now runners often ask Psyching Team members for pieces of tape. Taking advantage of these magical attributions, I instruct runners to hold the tape and listen carefully: They will be able to hear a message particular to them and their circumstances (Hays, 1990).

In the clinical setting of my office, I have at times used the tape as a transitional object, particularly if I will not be seeing clients for a while and they are experiencing distress. As with the runners, clients develop the phrase that is most appropriate for themselves (such as "let go" or "strength") and are also reminded of the connection they have with the therapist.

GOAL SETTING

Psychological skills training for athletes places considerable emphasis on goal setting and cognitive restructuring. Athletes with rigid win-lose orientations can be massively disappointed with a loss. Developing three levels of expectation (great, good enough, and tolerable) can allow the athlete to feel less anxious and more positively invested in the event.

> Initially, 22-year-old Sally felt that she would be an utter failure if she did not leave her moribund marriage by a certain date. An incest survivor and witness to her parents' troubled marriage, she fluctuated between precipitous action and anxious immobilization. As we examined her intentions, she began developing a more deliberate framework. Among other aspects of her planning, she widened her goal range: Even if she were not out of the house by the specified date, she would feel she was making progress if she had obtained a separate bank account, or at least had made and kept an initial legal appointment.

OTHER TECHNIQUES

A few other conceptual images and techniques to help trauma survivors, ones that cannot be neatly categorized, are also worth mentioning. As described earlier, improvements in athletic skill occur because of alterations in the FIT, the acronym that refers to changes in the frequency, intensity and time (duration) of practice. One can also use the concept of FIT to reflect changes in any behavioral or emotional symptom of PTSD, that is, whether it is more or less frequent, intense, or long. Clients find these measures easy to use for themselves. They also come to appreciate the ways in which change is multidimensional. For example, rage may still occur as often, but it may not be as intense as it had been or it may not last as long.

> After a number of weeks of good interpersonal contact, 35-year-old Toni, an anorexic incest survivor, spent time in a dissociated state one day during therapy. She fell into silence and seemed to have difficulty focusing her attention. Toward the end of the hour, after she had struggled to come back into the session, I expressed concern about our disconnection. Understanding FIT, she pointed out that she was dissociating in session much less frequently, was able to come back with less struggle, and that the disconnection had lasted a shorter period of time.

Questions of emotional safety are often present for survivors of sexual abuse. While under water, SCUBA divers use a hand signal to indicate to each other that a situation is under control (they touch thumb and forefinger together to indicate that everything is "okay"). Clients using this kinesthetic "anchor" or tactile symbol can remind themselves that in fact things are okay, that they are safe, and that the current situation is different from that of the trauma. It serves as reassurance, allows the development of a sense of self-trustworthiness, and reminds clients that they can comfort and sooth themselves (McCann & Pearlman, 1990).

PRACTITIONER RECOMMENDATIONS

This chapter has differed from most of the others in this section in that I have devoted much of it to explaining techniques with accompanying brief vignettes of practitioner applications. Rather than further describe the techniques, the recommendations I make here are directed toward their appropriate use.

In recommending exercise to trauma survivors, practitioners may want to be alert to and possibly address issues of physical or psychological safety, body image, and body awareness. For clients who are not accustomed to venturing with their bodies, the realm of exercise can become a safe place to work out concerns that in other contexts are more fraught with meaning.

Exercise may be most effective in moderating affect if it has the qualities described by Berger (1994; e.g., pleasing and enjoyable, aerobic or requiring rhythmical abdominal breathing, involving an absence of interpersonal competition, predictable or temporally and spatially certain, and of moderate intensity).

Some of the psychological skills techniques, such as arousal management, should be taught to any client experiencing heightened levels of arousal. Others, such as the pep cheer for concentration and focus, may be one of a number of techniques used at various points throughout therapy. Although certain techniques are fairly straight-forward, others, such as visualization, should only be undertaken by a therapist with skill and knowledge of both the technique and its uses for trauma survivors.

The adept practitioner individualizes techniques to the person and situation. Creative combining and interweaving of these methods can have an exponentiating effect. Affirmations, for example, often work better when accompanied by imagery. Imagery, in turn, is typically preceded by controlled breathing techniques. Because these tech-niques can be effective (i.e., powerful), practitioners will find it useful to obtain supervision or consult with peers regarding their use.

Healthy and Strong:
Exercise and Recovery From Medical Illness

14

At the 1995 APA convention, a colleague and I were out for an early run in Central Park. We were struck speechless as a young woman approached us. She was astoundingly thin. She walked rapidly, her right leg encased in a cast. Was she anorexic, driven to continue exercise despite injury? Alternatively, was exercise part of a rehabilitation program she was engaged in? Aware of the ways in which we were using exercise to prepare for the stresses of the day and to connect with each other, silently we wished her well in whatever stressors she was facing in her life.

The interrelation of exercise with illness, injury, and overuse is a complex one, and, as illustrated above, not always immediately apparent. In this chapter I review the ways in which exercise has mental benefits for those with medical illnesses. I address issues regarding the overuse of exercise in chapter 18.

Discussion

Sime's term *somatopsychic* (Sime, 1996) is especially apt when considering the mental benefits of exercise for those with physical illnesses. Exercise benefits have been noted with regard to heart disease, chronic obstructive pulmonary disease, irritable bowel syndrome, arthritis, menstrual cramps, back pain, sleep disorders, migraine headaches, and symptoms of AIDS (Sime, 1996). In addition to improving cardiopulmonary function, for example, exercise in cardiac rehabilitation potentially can serve to decrease anger and hostility, anxiety, and depression (Sime, 1996).

Noted here are investigations and programs addressing people with coronary difficulties, cancer, HIV and AIDS, and some of the invisible chronic illnesses, such as arthritis, lupus, and chronic fatigue syndrome.

The connections and pathways between coronary status, depression, and exercise are probably significant, but have not been explored. The level of depression may affect degree of self-care during cardiac rehabilitation, including exercise (Conn, Taylor, & Wiman, 1991). This suggests that practitioners may need to take into account the co-acting fatigue of myocardial infarction recovery and depression and carefully assess stage of change in order to maximize effective processes. A meta-analysis of 28 studies of the relationship between exercise and anxiety and depression in coronary patients found effect sizes, but these were smaller than those of psychotherapeutic interventions (Kugler, Seelbach, & Kruskemper, 1994). An experiment assessing the psychological impact of exercise training with or without relaxation therapy in myocardial infarct patients found that the addition of relaxation therapy significantly improved physical outcome and decreased anxiety (Van Dixhoorn, Duivenvoorden, Pool, & Verhage, 1990).

There is equivocal information regarding the relationship between exercise and cancer prevention. Most studies have shown that exercise serves a protective function (Pinto & Marcus, 1994), although some others have suggested no protection and a potential increased risk (Lerner, 1994). As with other investigations involving mind–body links, it may be in the common pathways that the effects are most pronounced. Depression, for example, is both a common precursor of and concomitant factor in cancer. If exercise affects depression, it may indirectly help prevent or modulate the development of a cancer.

There appear to be no research studies of the mental utility of exercise with people with already existing cancer (Lerner, 1994). However, the sense of action and hope conveyed by the annual North American fund-raising events known as the Race for the Cure speaks to at least a symbolic connection. More concretely, some programs of physical activity are designed specifically for people with cancer. Dragon boating and racing, involving 20 paddlers, a steerperson, and a drummer, has become popular in some Canadian cities among breast cancer survivors (Turner, 1998). The benefits for members of one group, Dragons Abreast, include camaraderie, acceptance, team cohesion, mastery, distraction, and physical exertion. One woman commented, "I already know they can't cure me, but I want to build my body back up, to have as normal a life as I can have. . . . [This is] the best therapy I could have" (Turner, 1998, p. L2).

As he journeyed to the end of his life, increasingly impeded by prostate cancer, running guru and writer George Sheehan, MD, wrote a final book reflecting on the meaning of physical activity in his life. Formerly introverted, socially isolated, and highly competitive, he wrote:

> Cancer has its rewards, and one of them has been finding other values in my running. My therapy has put me far back in the race. When I come to the finish line there are few runners behind me. Competition, and the trophies that go with it, no longer attracts me. For the first time the most important thing about running has become my fellow runners. (1996, p. 59)

Although there have been very few studies of the effect of exercise with HIV-positive patients, those that have been done suggest a markedly positive benefit. LaPerriere and others (LaPerriere, Fletcher, Antoni, Klimas, Ironson, & Schneiderman, 1991) conducted a 10-week study with gay men randomly assigned to aerobic exercise or assessment-only control. Participants' levels of anxiety and depression were assessed 72 hours prior to and following notification of their HIV status. Control group members who were seropositive experienced significantly greater increases in both anxiety and depression than did either seropositive exercisers or those in either group who were seronegative. In a study of physical self-efficacy, mood, and life satisfaction, 33 HIV-infected men were randomly assigned to aerobic training, anaerobic weight training, or a control (stretching and flexibility) group (Lox, McAuley, & Tucker, 1995). Both exercise groups experienced improved perceived physical ability, increased positive mood and life satisfaction, and decreased negative mood over the course of the study. Results were in the opposite direction on nearly all measures for members of the control group. No negative effects for exercise were reported (Lox, McAuley, & Tucker, 1995). Further studies, Lox, McAuley, and Tucker suggested, should broaden the populations studied (e.g., women and youths) and examine dose-response issues.

> **Mostly I create, write, go into this world of ideas which is so magical in that it has no relation to the troubles of my world or personal life. Sometimes I space out on the scenery, especially if I go skiing alone. Other times I tune into the power of my physical self. But I always go somewhere great and seem to know how to get there if it does not happen when I don the shoes or goggles or head out the door or down the lap lane.**
>
> **44-year-old female psychologist with chronic medical condition**

Invisible chronic illnesses, "diseases that are characterized by chronicity and symptoms that are not externally manifested" (Donoghue & Siegel, 1992), include arthritis, irritable bowel syndrome, multiple sclerosis, Crohn's disease, fibromyalgia, lupus erythematosus, chronic fatigue syndrome, and chronic pain. Although vastly different illnesses, they have commonalities of variable illness course; frequently being nonobservable, especially during sometimes extended phases of remission; and being characterized at least in part by subjective rather than objective symptoms.

A 4-month aerobic exercise program for a wide age range of participants with rheumatoid arthritis resulted in significant reduction in depression and improvement in measures of quality of life, with no negative physical effects (Perlman et al., 1990). This study was designed to assess the relative effects of exercise and behavior therapy on patients' self-report of pain and disability from chronic low back pain, and compared behavioral, exercise, and behavioral plus exercise treatments with a wait list control group. Mildly depressed and disabled before treatment, patients in the behavioral plus exercise combination described greatest satisfaction, followed by those in the exercise alone group, and then the behavioral program. Long term (6 and 12 months posttreatment) there was no statistically significant difference among the three interventions with regard to levels of pain and disability.

Approximately 131,000 people in the United States between the ages of 15 and 65 are afflicted with systemic lupus erythematosus (SLE), a chronic inflammatory disease resulting from immunoregulatory disturbances of genetic, hormonal and environmental factors that affects women nine times more often than men (Braden, McGlone, & Pennington, 1993). Although the experimental design was flawed in some ways, participants in an SLE self-help course reported improved and sustained self-care activities, including exercise, as well as decreased depression and increased enabling skills (perceived ability to manage adversity), following didactic training that focused on these issues.

> Evy, a 22-year-old college graduate, sought treatment because she wanted to start exercising again. An active basketball player throughout high school, she had developed chronic fatigue syndrome during college. Although her physician indicated by her senior year that she was physically recovered, Evy found that when she exercised, she became extremely anxious that any tiredness she experienced was an indicator of the return of her illness. In turn, she became even more anxious, vigilant, and immobile.
>
> Seeking to help decrease her anxiety, I taught her deep breathing and encouraged her to use a cue relaxation word,

using her thumbnail as focus object. I suggested that she practice this three times a day. Additionally, I suggested she develop a reasonable plan of exercise and actively begin counteracting any thoughts that she was ill.

Evy decided to use walking as her form of exercise, even though she found it uninteresting. She started by walking 15 minutes a day. Still anxious, she decided to stay near home to reduce her fear.

Over the next few weeks, she gradually increased the length of her walks. As she continued bored with the form of exercise but motivated to resolve her anxiety, she became more ready to become venturesome. We discussed the importance of FIT, and she greatly appreciated Csikszentmihalyi's pictorial representation (1990, p. 74) of "flow" as a continuous, synergistic balance between challenge and skill. By maintaining this balance, she could avoid the alternative potential pitfalls of either anxiety or boredom.

Evy was very proud when she bought her first pair of athletic shoes in 4 years. She began feeling as if she were regaining some of her lost self. Ready to branch out on her own after five sessions, we discussed her plans, possible relapse issues, and reemphasized the importance of gradual change.

Practitioner Recommendations

The need for coordination between practitioner and other health care providers is of course particularly critical with patients who are medically ill. Patients need to obtain appropriate services and practitioners need to not step over the bounds of competence or role. Psychotherapists often need to interact with medical personnel, including physician specialists, physical therapists, occupational therapists, or exercise physiologists.

There are a number of role relationship possibilities for the psychotherapist in this team approach. In addition to serving as the primary psychotherapist, the practitioner also may be in an excellent position to train or consult with other personnel in psychological management of the patient.

Exercise among people with illness provides the opportunity for considerable individual self-assessment as the patient becomes part of the treatment team (Heil, Wakefield, & Reed, 1998) and begins assessing the type and FIT of exercise that works best. Internal appraisal can be used to develop clarity concerning the best type and timing of exercise. Clients can keep a log that identifies exercise type, intensity, physical symptoms, and mood changes. This type of record, if kept over time and reviewed, can prove informative. What may seem, initially, to be unpredictable in terms of effect on fatigue, for example, may over time become an expectable and thus tolerable pattern.

To the extent that the person can tolerate exercise physiologically, from a psychological perspective the type of exercise that may be most effective may be suggested by their psychological symptoms. Yoga, for example, may be especially useful for anxiety, stress management and relaxation; brisk walking or running may be especially useful to alleviate depression.

Oxymorons and Stereotypes: 15
Exercise and Diversity Issues

I nstead of focusing on particular clinical syndromes, in this chapter I draw attention to generic and specific issues regarding barriers and opportunities in the use of exercise in therapy with certain diverse populations. The perspective I take here is that it is the socially constructed understandings that are brought to the relationship between people in these population categories in relation to the use of exercise that are of significance. This dynamic refers both to the client's own understanding and approach as well as that of the practitioner. The particular groups about which some information is available include (in descending order of information) women, gay men and lesbians, and people of color. The lack of discussion of other issues of considerable importance, such as socioeconomic status or disability in relation to exercise, let alone interactions among these various groups, reflects an absence of research information (Gill, 1995; Physical activity, 1997) rather than an unintended omission of these groups in this discussion.

Discussion of exercise in cultural context appears almost inextricably interwoven with sport in our society. And "sport is more sexist, heterosexist, and homophobic than the larger society" (Gill, 1995, p. 225). It may be more racist as well. Because exercise may occur within organized sport, in this chapter focused on issues of socially constructed meaning, I include more reference to the athletic setting than I do in many of the other chapters.

There is another layer of cultural context as well: The athletic environment may be viewed as culturally distinct in some ways (Cogan, 1998; Lamont-Mills & Pretty, 1997). In exploring diversity of any type it is critical to strike a balance between acknowledging social and cultural influences that may be salient while not making sweeping generalizations based on stereotypic beliefs and information (Cogan & Petrie, 1996b). In an effort not to make alpha errors that magnify difference, it is important not to swing too far in the alternate direction of beta errors that minimize difference (Oglesby & Hill, 1993). As with all work with human beings, recognizing and valuing individual differences is critical. Either explicitly or implicitly, the therapist will want to address those differences that exist between helper and client (Petrie, 1998).

Drawing on the diversity literature, Mooney (1993) delineated a multicultural perspective for the athletic environment. This perspective addresses situations in which one is working with those not like oneself along some important dimensions of self and identity, for example sex, sexual orientation, or ethnicity. Therapists supporting clients' exercise behavior yet whose sex, sexual orientation, or ethnicity differs from their clients will be well advised to have the following characteristics:

- cultural self-awareness and sensitivity;
- openness to and respect for differing value systems;
- tolerance for ambiguity;
- willingness to learn with and from clients;
- genuine concern for people with differing value systems;
- awareness of one's own assumptions, values, or biases; and
- knowledge about the unique characteristics of the group with which one is working.

Women, Sports and Exercise: Overcoming the Oxymoron

In shining a spotlight on women in relation to exercise, the magnification of difference reflects gender (that is, psychosocial construction) rather than sex differences per se. These differences are so embedded in all of our cultural experiences that, for example, it may take many readings of the respective newsletters of APA's Division of Women in Psychology (Division 35) and Division of Men and Masculinity (Divison 51) to note that in the former there are never references to sport or exercise, whether as analogy or as activity, yet in contrast there are always at least a few in the latter.

The history of our knowledge about women and sport, like that of much scholarly research, has been that of generalizing from the experience of male sport participants to all sport participants (Bredemeier et al., 1991; Cogan & Petrie, 1996b; Duda, 1991). Further, most research that has been conducted has focused on performance, competitive sport, and quantitative rather than qualitative studies (Duda, 1991; Lenskyj, 1990). These research biases are especially unfortunate in sport, since the socialized experience of men and women has been so dramatically different. Sport has been veridical for males, but often an oxymoron for females.

Traditionally, the physical meaning of gender has been strikingly different. Masculinity has been associated with energy, strength, and motion, whereas femininity has been associated with quiescence, limitation, and protection. Body image issues for men focus on size and strength; female concerns relate to appearance (weight and slenderness) (Rindskopf & Gratch, 1982). Whereas boys consider that excess weight relates to muscle, girls attribute it to fat. And if men want to lose weight, they typically will increase exercise, whereas women will start to diet. A further erosion occurs when appearance is the definition of value: The capacity to age gracefully or with a sense of competence becomes undermined.

The early 1970s saw the beginning of the most recent wave of women's engagement in physical activity. The women's movement, Title IX (1972), and the development of the Women's Sports Foundation (1974) created an atmosphere for a reclamation of women's bodies and a concomitant surge in interest in understanding women's experience in sport and exercise. Reflecting that energy at a popular level, *WomenSport* magazine, now *Women's Sports + Fitness*, was founded in 1974. Yet even today, girls and women, compared with boys and men, tend to be more sedentary and less involved in physical activity, as well as less engaged in organized, competitive sport (Duda, 1991). And there has been comparatively little research or writing about gender issues in applied sport psychology (Gill, 1995).

There is a paradox: Exercise is especially valuable for women, yet underappreciated by this same group. Female gender is one of the predictors of lack of exercise initiation (Dishman, 1994a). Lack of modeling, lack of social supports from friends or family, and a culturally prescribed attitude of selflessness are further barriers. Each of these issues is the direct obverse of those factors critical to the adoption of exercise (Sallis et al., 1992).

PHYSICAL BENEFITS OF EXERCISE FOR WOMEN

In addition to the many physical benefits of exercise for the population as a whole, for example, decreased risk for coronary heart disease,

> I alternate days between treadmill and weights—would love to swim, but it doesn't help osteoporosis! When I swam, I thought more creatively. With other forms of exercise, I tune out.
>
> **52-year-old female psychologist**

hypertension, and colon cancer (United States Department of Health and Human Services, 1996), exercise also impacts more specifically female-related concerns such as premenstrual syndrome (PMS) menopause, osteoporosis, breast cancer, muscle mass loss, and weight management.

In a scathing critique of the prescription of psychotropic medications for premenstrual dysphoria, Prior, Gill, and Vigna (1995) encouraged instead the recommendation of aerobic exercise. They noted decreased fluid retention and breast tenderness after a 3-month program of mildly increasing exercise, and decreased mood symptoms after 6 months of minimal regular physical activity. They commented:

> Why test an expensive drug when an inexpensive change in lifestyle, free of side effects and with positive effects on cardiovascular disease and the risk of osteoporosis, can be expected to provide benefit. . . . Science thinks it must rescue women from their bodies . . . more evidence of the negative view this culture holds of women and their physiology. (p. 1152)

Steege and Blumenthal (1993) compared the effects of randomly assigned aerobic exercise and (anaerobic) strength training on PMS symptoms of 23 healthy premenopausal women (45–55). Measured at baseline and following 3 months of exercise participation, they found that both types of exercise served to reduce some PMS symptoms. Aerobic exercise appeared to decrease depressive symptoms as well as more of the PMS symptoms. Preliminary findings in the Study of Women's Health Across the Nation (SWAN) suggest that, regardless of ethnicity, menopausal women who report getting less physical activity describe more estrogen-related and somatic symptoms (DeAngelis, 1997). In contrast, exercise appears associated with decreased severity of hot flashes, although it is not clear whether this is a direct effect or mediated through the mechanism of diaphragmatic breathing (Barbach, 1994).

PSYCHOLOGICAL BENEFITS OF EXERCISE FOR WOMEN

As I described in previous chapters, exercise is effective in the management of psychological conditions that disproportionately affect women, such as depression and posttraumatic stress disorder (McGrath et al., 1990). Additionally, physical fitness training can result in a resocialization of body perceptions for women and girls:

body experiences which are not traditionally feminine. When exercise is strenuous, appearance is deemphasized. The sweatiness, labored breathing, tangled hair and facial grimaces that accompany hard physical exertion become part of the everyday experience. A new sense of body strength is gained as muscles replace fat and are capable of more and more work. Body competence is discovered as the first continuous mile or miles is achieved. Physical risk-taking occurs and pain becomes a sign of progress rather than a signal to stop. Even clothing becomes increasingly functional. Although improved muscle tone and, often, weight loss affect appearance in an external sense, the changes described are primarily internal. A woman can begin to appreciate her body for its power and function, variables over which she has an exceedingly reasonable degree of control. (Rindskopf & Gratch, 1982, pp. 20f.)

Rindskopf and Gratch developed a 10-week program of group walking and running plus group psychotherapy in which clients' body satisfaction was renewed. "The locus of healing and eventually the locus for prevention are returned to the individual woman. The health she restores is a strong, realistic one which ages gracefully, and is a steady reminder of her own competence" (Rindskopf & Gratch 1982, p. 25).

WOMEN AND SOCIABILITY

The social support and connection that many exercise programs provide is an important aspect of exercise adherence for many women, with their sensitivity to relationship. At the same time, for others it is the opportunity for legitimate disconnection that is particularly valued. Johnsgard suggests that one of the functions of exercise is to regulate social distance, "to satisfy needs for privacy or social contact" (1989, p. 38). Women overburdened with child care responsibilities or the social commerce of life, for example, may experience legitimate solitude as a sought-after luxury.

> Having wrested a few precious moments from the demands of child care and work care, Rebecca felt a special sense of triumph one day when the swimming pool at her gym was nearly empty. Paraphrasing Virginia Woolf, she appreciated having "a lane of my own."

GENDER-DEVELOPMENTAL INTERACTIONS IN RELATION TO SPORT AND EXERCISE

Girlhood and Adolescence

Even at an early age, gender role stereotyping and socialization result in marked differences between boys and girls in their attitudes about and involvement in sports (Cogan & Petrie, 1996b; Eccles & Harold, 1991). By grade 1, despite essentially comparable skills, girls feel significantly less competent in sport than do boys. They also are significantly less invested in the sport domain than are boys, and see sports as less important than other, academic, areas (Eccles & Harold, 1991).

One might anticipate that 25 years of experience and opportunity since the passage of Title IX should offset cultural biases and stereotypes, yet the impact and effectiveness of this federal legislation continues to be mixed (Duncan, 1997). Research in the 1970s suggested that women athletes experienced role conflict. Subsequently, criticism of the role conflict literature suggested that societal problems were being located within the individual. The issue is a "male referent model (i.e., athleticism = maleness) which does not capture or celebrate the potential realities of female participation in sport" (Allison, 1991, p. 59). Although role conflict may still be prevalent as the century ends, women may be increasingly able to resolve the disjuncture in ways that can allow them to be female and athletes. A high school basketball player, for example, said: "The court is where you can be all those things we're not supposed to be: aggressive, cocky, strong" (Blais, 1995, p. 229). In another example: during intensive interviews, collegiate women athletes recently reported significant role conflict (Bacon, 1997), yet they reacted with anger rather than withdrawal or shame. This response suggested that one of the net effects of increased female participation in sport may be a decreased sense of internalized role conflict, even if some sturdy vestiges of external role conflict remain.

In the past few years, research has focused on the ways in which exercise may have an important impact on the lives of adolescent girls. A recent report by the President's Council on Physical Fitness and Sports (Physical activity, 1997) summarized much of this research. Although physical activity generally is associated with improved self-esteem and body image, the relationship is not uniformly straightforward for adolescent athletes, especially those involved in sports in which weight or appearance are relevant elements (Wiese-Bjornstal, 1997). Among White girls, athletes have lower school dropout rates and are more positively disposed toward the sciences than their nonathlete peers (Duncan, 1997). In regard to two major clinical issues for adolescent girls, depression and posttraumatic stress disorder, exercise therapy may offer a cost-effective treatment alternative or adjunct to traditional psychotherapy or antidepressant drugs, both of which are not predictably as effective for adolescents as they are for adults (Greenberg & Oglesby, 1997).

The interaction of exercise and bone mass is important, complex, and perhaps age-related. Although on the one hand, early exercise patterns can assist the development of bone mass, young women engaged in continual strenuous exercise are at higher risk for the "female athlete triad"—amenorrhea, disordered eating, and osteoporosis (Freedson & Bunker, 1997). In later years, however, the value of weight-bearing exercise or resistance training for the maintenance of bone mineral density and the prevention of osteoporosis has been well established (Crandall, 1986). The specific mechanisms are still being explored, as well as the intriguing question of whether exercise can serve as an osteogenic stimulus, that is, actually increase bone mass (Barbach, 1994; De Souza, Arce, Nulsen, & Puhl, 1994).

Adult and Aging Women

I had been passionate about dance when I was much younger, and assumed it was for a certain sort of youthful, lithe body. Six months ago I joined an intergenerational dance group, and I am now regularly rehearsing and performing with them.

Exercise keeps me aware of my body in a very realistic way. I know what my body can do and what it cannot do. I know that I can improve my flexibility and strength through yoga and relax it through tai chi and yoga.

We get hung up on how our bodies look rather than what our bodies can do. What I am interested in learning about through this new dance experience is the aesthetic of the aging body, learning to give up some of the expectations that women have about their bodies.

68-year-old female psychologist

Even more than adults in general, older adults and older women in particular tend not to participate in any kind of regular physical activity. "Throughout the life span, women are less active than their male counterparts, so that by late life, only a small minority are adequately exercising to benefit their health and well-being" (Cousins, 1996, p. 131).

Using Maehr and Braskamp's theory of personal investment—goals predict adherence—Gill and Overdorf (1994) suggested that exercise programs should be structured differently as a function of relevant incentives at various ages. In a study of 272 women aged 18 to 60 who were regular exercisers, younger women (under 31) focused more on weight management, whereas older women (over 51) focused increasingly on the physical and mental health benefits, social interaction, and stress reduction and mastery effects of exercise. Elderly women may exaggerate risks of exercise, underestimate their physical abilities, believe that exercise need decreases with age, lack appropriate role models, and lack knowledge concerning the health benefits of exercise.

PRACTITIONER RECOMMENDATIONS

Gender role socialization affects all of us. Psychotherapists, whether men or women, are not immune to the cultural isomorphism of (straight) men and sports—and, by extension, exercise. Psychotherapists thus may be less inclined to think about exercise as a treatment alternative or adjunct for female clients. If one of the main purposes of this book is to encourage psychotherapists to consider exercise for their clients, then this chapter underscores the utility of exercise for female clients in particular.

Women raised in the pre-Title IX era may be less likely to have a strong history of competitive sport to build on. There can be some advantages to the lack of sport domain value. If or when women do start exercising, they may not have as many ghosts to fight as men often do. There may be fewer old memories to play off of, fewer impossible-to-attain expectations of the self, and less identity attachment to one's own exercise as compared with that of others. If there are types of exercise a woman was involved with or wanted to do as a child, these may be particularly compelling and empowering as she sets out to increase her own sense of competence. An attitude of curiosity can be helpful, as well as an exploration of the most salient opportunities for or barriers to exercise.

A number of studies have noted the value of weight and strength training in enhancing adolescent girls' and women participants' self-concept and body image (Fisher & Thompson, 1994; Gill, 1995; Wiese-Bjornstal, 1997). At the same time, women may feel daunted by male-dominated weight rooms in health clubs as well as unfamiliar equipment. The therapist should be alert to clients' possible need for assistance in problem solving, whether it is obtaining specific instruction in equipment use or finding social support.

Issues involving role modeling, social support for activity, self-efficacy for activity, and taking time for women's own needs should all be addressed directly. Often, as illustrated in various vignettes throughout this book, exercise may be a concrete opportunity to resolve some of these generic life issues.

No reliable information exists regarding the frequency with which female as compared with male mental health practitioners make recommendations of exercise to their clients. The particular gender pairing of therapist and client may be a factor in exercise recommendation, although there is no substantiated information in this regard. As with exercising with clients, I would expect that such advice from male therapists may be received by women clients as anticipated, albeit paternalistic. Response to female therapists' recommendations may be somewhat more variable. Although female therapists may be perceived by their female clients as role models, there is also a potential down side: A client might reify her exercising therapist even more than occurs in the course of treatment, with the possibility of distancing the relationship or diminishing the client's own motivation. Discussion of these issues can turn them into opportunities for learning.

Sexual Orientation

DISCUSSION

There is no information to suggest that exercise issues are different in any specific way based on sexual orientation. However, organized sport, like the armed forces, is one of the last bastions of rigid homonegativity, and is compulsively masculinized and heterosexist (Andersen, Butki, & Heyman, 1996). A survey of college students' attitudes toward and perceptions of lesbians and gay men yielded a main effect for gender and athletic status. Male students and athletes expressed more homophobic attitudes and perceptions than did female students or nonathletes (Andersen, Butki, & Heyman, 1996).

Men and athletes experience a direct threat with regard to women's engagement in sport, as expressed in the title of Mariah Burton Nelson's (1994) book, *The Stronger Women Get, the More Men Love Football*. From there, it is a quick step to homonegativity, embedded in which is an underlying assumption that to be male in sport equates with heterosexuality, yet to be female in sport implies being lesbian (Gill, 1995).

> By discrediting all women in sport as lesbians, men can rest assured that their territory is not being invaded by "real" women after all; by mobilizing societal prejudices against homosexuality, they may be able to keep the number of women involved in sport to a safe minimum; by creating an atmosphere of danger, they can, through innuendo, effectively prevent individual women from wanting to be involved in sport; and by keeping women from sport, they keep women from discovering the joy and power of their own physicality and they remove a potential arena for the development of female solidarity. Thus the norms of compulsory heterosexuality accomplish hegemonic closure. (Birrell, 1988)

Gay, lesbian, and bisexual athletes face the same concerns as other gay, lesbian, and bisexual people in our culture, with some potential additional issues as well (Cogan & Petrie, 1996b). In the past number of years, a few well-known athletes (e.g., Martina Navratilova, Greg Louganis) have "come out." Yet the general lack of role modeling of gay athletes of either sex can result in personal doubt and identity conflicts, extreme anxiety about being "outed," perhaps especially for men (Cogan & Petrie, 1996b), or a reactive, hypermasculine, high-risk persona (Waddell & Schaap, 1996).

Following the gay liberation of the 1970s, major metropolitan areas saw the development of a hypermasculine sexuality within gay culture (Levine, 1998). Intensive body building at specific gyms and athletic attire became an intrinsic aspect of the social life within gay "ghettos." "The cliques, crowds, and circuit provided the men with commonality, companionship, community, and contacts" (Levine, 1998, p. 53).

In any system with majority and minority cultures, the marginalized group faces the options of becoming exclusive or inclusive, whether through isolation, assimilation, adaptation, or incorporation. Levine described the development of the identity of the "gay clone," a kind of cooptation of the majority definitions of masculinity. Alternatively, the Gay Games, a quadrennial event begun in 1982 by Olympic decathlete Tom Waddell, were designed to be inclusive, not only with regard to sexual orientation, but race, gender, age, athleticism, and nationality as well (Waddell & Schaap, 1996).

Therapy with lesbian or gay high school and collegiate athletes often involves work on gender identity and guilt in addition to the presenting problem. Socialized in the isomorphism of sport and heterosexuality, the dilemma of gay men will be how to be able to be athletes and at the same time, gay. For women, the dilemma may be how to be athletic and female (Heyman, 1987). Heyman described therapy with these athletes as "a long, slow process, filled with denials, reaction for-

> I was a sickly kid, the epitome of the 90 lb weakling. I hated gym class, in part, because of my general lack of competence but also because I was often harassed in the locker room by classmates and in class by coaches. (Perhaps they knew I was gay before I did.) I gave up on sports in junior high school afer being ridiculed by a coach for being the last one to finish a 1 mile run.
>
> I took some aerobics classes in college but it wasn't until much later that I found running. At first, running was just a way to deal with stress and to clear my head after work. At the age of 37, I joined the frontrunners, a gay running group and began to increase my stamina. Two years later, I finished my first marathon.
>
> It wasn't until I trained for the marathon that I began to experience the physical and psychological benefits of running longer distances. The distances and commitment required in training for a marathon changed the way I felt about my body. For the first time in my life, I liked the way my body felt and looked.
>
> **40-year-old male psychologist**

mations, and even acting out behaviors." He also commented on the differences between gay male and female athletes. Because of the stereotype of heterosexuality, questions may not be raised about male athletes' sexual orientation, even if they do not date (women or men). Women who do not date may be presumptively cast as lesbian. On the other hand, Heyman suggested that there was less tension within women's sports teams with lesbian members, and more support through visible lesbian communities.

The lack of tolerance for homosexuality within the athletic environment appears not to have abated over time (Andersen, Butki, & Heyman, 1996). Today, male athletes' homonegativity is further compounded and perhaps cloaked by concerns about HIV and AIDS.

PRACTITIONER RECOMMENDATIONS

In order for the therapist to work effectively with a gay or lesbian population, his or her own issues with regard to sexual orientation need to be addressed (Cogan & Petrie, 1996b; Rotella & Murray, 1991). The heterosexual practitioner working with gay men or lesbians may need to increase self-awareness not only about attitudes and beliefs about sexual orientation in general but also about the ways in which sexual orientation interacts with the sporting or exercise environment. This can serve as an opportunity for increased self-reflection and self-awareness.

The lesbian or gay male practitioner working with gay and lesbian athletes or clients in relation to exercise should use the shared identification to attend to the client's needs rather than overidentify and experience boundary slippage. As in other areas of practice, the practitioner should consider the client's needs in deciding whether or not to indicate her or his sexual orientation (Cabaj, 1996).

The sexual orientation of the individual psychotherapy client may or may not be relevant to that person's experience of individual exercise activities. In contrast, the client engaged in group activities and in organized or competitive sports faces the potential, if not the actuality, of encountering aspects of homonegativity.

Ethnicity

DISCUSSION

Few studies have examined exercise in relation to ethnicity. In terms of physical health, this interaction is important to explore, since Blacks are at higher risk than their White counterparts for hypertension, diabetes, or obesity, yet have lower-than-average levels of physical activity (Airhihenbuwa, Kumanyika, Agurs, & Lowe, 1995; Klesges, DeBon, & Meyers, 1996). In one of the few experimental studies to specifically control for race as well as gender, Rejeski, Thompson, Brubaker, and Miller (1992) found that acute aerobic exercise of 40 minutes duration was an effective buffer to psychosocial stressors. In light of the increased risk for hypertension among Blacks, and the statistically higher resting systolic blood pressure among this group of 24 Black as compared with 24 White women 25–40 years old, this information was especially important.

> Referred for psychotherapy by her physician in part because of chronic stress that potentially was interfering with her fertility, 38-year-old Angela, a Caribbean immigrant, was simultaneously eager for emotional relief yet interpersonally extremely cautious. Initial treatment recommendations included encouragement of journal writing for disclosure to herself, if not her therapist, diaphragmatic breathing, and exercise. In the process of physical recovery from a miscarriage some months earlier, Angela had discontinued playing tennis, an activity that she loved, and had not thought about since. Needing only slight encouragement, she joined a new league. She experienced immediate satisfaction and pride in her skill, as well as some decrease in stress.

The interaction among various demographic characteristics, including age, education, socioeconomic status, and particular ethnicity is of considerable interest and offers many intriguing possibilities. Surveys are just beginning to be developed and a clear pattern has yet to emerge. For example, in a recent study (Jaffee & Lutter, 1995), 44% of Black female adolescents, as compared with 33% of Native American and 32% of White girls, reported having a good body image. They also were markedly more likely to consider themselves more attractive, liked the way they looked, and felt competent about their bodies. At the same time, certain cultures may be less tolerant of students who challenge gender-stereotyped behavior, and girls of color tend to be less involved in intramural sports than their White peers (Duncan, 1997). High school athletes' attributions of success and failure may interact with gender, number of years of experience, and ethnicity (Morgan, Griffin, & Heyward, 1996). Comparing African American, Anglo, Hispanic, and Native American students, attributional differences are apparent regarding perceived social mobility, cultural values associated with group and family, cooperation, knowledge and tradition, and present vs. future time orientation. The experience of success and failure is culturally and situationally, as well as individually, determined.

Through focus group interviews of 53 participants stratified by age, and for older people, sex and socioeconomic status, Airhihenbuwa and colleagues (1995) found that African Americans of limited economic resources, themselves involved in physical labor, equated their work life with physical activity. They felt they had little available leisure time and considered rest, as a means of compensating for their labor, more important than exercise. Exercise was perceived as a physical stressor.

There is a dearth of information on Black women, and even less on the athletic experiences of other women of color such as Chicanas, Asian women, and Native American women (Birrell, 1988; Cogan & Petrie, 1996b; Hall, 1998). Whereas 58% of women in the United States are reportedly inactive, 65% of minority women are inactive (Pinto, 1994). Reviewing African American women's use of exercise for therapeutic purposes, Hall (1998) suggested that the therapist needs to consider the client's attitude toward therapy, exercise, and physical health; socioeconomic status; diagnosis; support system; styles of coping with stress; attitude toward self-care; body image; and exposure to realistic role models who exercise. Hall reported that African American women describe themselves as "softly strong," and thus some of the role conflicts around femininity and activity experienced by White women may be less conflictual for them. Health concerns (vs. appearance) and social opportunities may be salient factors in exercise motivation for African Americans (Airhihenbuwa et al., 1995; Hall, 1998). Taking into account class issues as well as the cultural value of interconnectedness, Hall suggested that low-income African American women may find group activities, such as dance and walking, more attractive and accessible than weight training, swimming, or cycling. Airhihenbuwa and colleagues' (1995) focus groups came to similar conclusions.

PRACTITIONER RECOMMENDATIONS

Generalization and specific practitioner recommendations are perilous at best, given the minimal information available concerning issues of race and exercise in psychotherapy or the interacting effects of race, sex, orientation, and class. The information provided by Hall is a good starting place. The therapist needs to be aware of the implicit assumptions, biases, and stereotypes about race and ethnicity that she or he may bring to the treatment relationship.

Having Fun:
Exercise Across the Life Span

16

E xercise has different meanings for people at various ages and stages of development. As with the previous chapter, I focus here not on psychological syndromes per se, but the interaction of exercise and age in regard to mental health and well-being.

The core values of sportsmanship, leadership, and cooperation are often cited as essentials of youth sports, yet there is little substantiation for this assertion. Weiss (1995) notes that "positive self-perceptions, intrinsic motivation, enjoyment, positive attitude toward the value of physical activity, ability to cope with stress, and sportspersonlike attitudes" (p. 42) are not inherent to children's competitive sport. As in other situations and settings, modeling of values and attitudes is most effective if it is specific. Similarly, consultation with parents and coaches needs to be directed toward shaping programs and experiences to maximize the likelihood of these emotional and attitudinal outcomes (Smith & Smoll, 1996; Weiss, 1995).

The 60-year tradition of therapeutic work with children ranges from play therapy with board games or enactments to activity therapy such as shooting baskets while talking. Adolescence, a time for identity formation, is a time of high stress that may be buffered by engagement in physical activity. There is a vast amount of information concerning college student athletes, although very little about non-sports-related exercise among this population. Likewise, most of the information concerning adults focuses on competitive athletes. Among older people, increasingly, programs are being designed to take into account the mental as well as physical benefits of exercise. Because of the lack of research information concerning young adulthood and midlife, specifically in relation to exercise and mental health, I do not describe these groups in detail here.

Children and Exercise

The cartoon strip "Cathy" illustrates the contrast between child and adult experiences of exercise: A delighted child runs among playground equipment in a picture entitled "The Gym, Ages 1–10." In contrast, "The Gym, Rest of Life," shows Cathy in anxious tears as she stands at the door of a fitness center with a sign posted: New Thigh Machines. In the six pictures that follow, Cathy and a friend watch her friend's daughter run, go up and down steps, lift buckets of sand, ride her bike, and then beg to go swimming. Observing her, the two adults discuss the work that they have created of exercise, asking plaintively, "Why can't it still be fun for us?"

DISCUSSION

Infants and children learn about the world through movement and interaction. The challenge for adults is to support and enhance those attributes both for current physical and psychological development and for later pleasure in physical activity (Biddle, 1993). Programs for children need to take into account a variety of developmental factors, including chronological, developmental, cognitive, physical, and emotional maturity (Crandall, 1986). Although each program will vary by sport, skill level, and individual, it has been suggested that developmentally, the primary focus from ages 6–10 should be to create an interest in sports in general, have fun, and learn basic skills; from 11–14, to increase versatility and technical skill; and from 15–18, to increase training intensity, competition, and specialization (Crandall, 1986).

In a poignantly descriptive study of 380 children, 8–12 years old, Rose, Larkin, and Berger (1994) noted marked discrepancies between objectively poorly coordinated students and their more well-coordinated peers. Regardless of sex, the clumsy children perceived themselves as receiving significantly less social support from their peers (classmates and close friend), teachers, and parents than did their more physically skilled classmates. Further, "the clumsy children had lower perceptions of close friendship than their well-coordinated peers. . . . A picture of loneliness and isolation in poorly coordinated children is apparent from these findings" (p. 20). To compound matters further, the well-coordinated children perceived themselves as receiving significantly higher support from both parents and teachers than did those less skilled. Whether this was an actual or perceived halo effect, it does suggest that there is a complex synergistic interaction between physical coordination, social network and comfort, and self-confidence.

At the same time, exercise has been found to enhance self-esteem, particularly among those most at risk, such as children with emotional disturbance, retardation, economic disadvantage, or perceptual handicaps (Horn & Claytor, 1993). Kern, Koegel, and Dunlap (1984) reported that after 15 min of jogging, stereotyped behavior such as hand and arm flopping and body rocking decreased in autistic children. Shipman (1984) described a 12-week program of long, slow distance running for 45 min, four times per week among residential and day patients in a psychiatric program. Naturalistic effects included spontaneous comments from teachers, who noted improved peer interactions and self-confidence, and greater calmness. An increase in positive parental engagement also occurred. There was a direct correlation between amount run and reduction in medication, especially for psychostimulants. The half-life of this treatment method appeared short-lived, however: When they stopped running, a number of the study participants "regressed in all areas of behavior."

A meta-analytic review of the relationship between exercise and disruptive behavior among various populations (children and adults, emotionally disturbed, physically disabled, conduct disordered, or developmentally disabled) concluded that antecedent (that is, noncontingent) exercise "is effective in reducing a variety of disruptive behaviors across a variety of populations (Allison, Faith, & Franklin, 1995, p. 297). In particular, greater effects were found in relation to hyperactive subjects and with nonaerobic exercise.

Obesity in childhood is an increasing problem. Twice as many children are currently overweight as there were in the 1960s. Obesity is represented dispropor-

> A few years ago, I worked at a private boarding school. We had children from all walks of life and from several countries. Some of the children were from abusive homes, some had emotional disorders, and one had recently lost a parent to a sudden illness. I found that a good friendly exhausting game of basketball or soccer helped the students wind down. After the games, the students would be able to open up and talk, cry, etc., because they had spent so much time on the court. They also told me that they felt more comfortable talking to me because I had played with them.
>
> **27-year-old female
> psychology graduate student**

tionately among the urban poor, some ethnic groups, and those with disabilities (Freedson & Bunker, 1997). And obese children tend to be inactive. Epstein (1992) suggests that two homeostatic implications follow. First, inactivity competes with activity. Lower levels of activity and lower levels of fitness interact. Second, much of that inactivity involves watching television, which itself is often an occasion for eating, food preoccupation, enticing advertisements of high calorie and low nutrition foods, and distorted understanding of the relationship between food intake and weight. Although emphasizing the importance of decreased caloric intake, Epstein encourages the development of an active lifestyle, useful not only as a complement to decreased intake but also the maintenance of lowered body weight.

Obese children may find walking a more reasonable and acceptable exercise method than running for two reasons, Epstein (1992) suggests. The necessary component of exercise for weight loss is caloric expenditure rather than intensity, and intense exercise may be associated with decreased compliance. Some successful projects have used family-based procedures, involving parents as well as children. Such programs create an opportunity for systemic lifestyle change and healthy family interaction.

Parental engagement in children's exercise and sport behavior is a double-edged sword, simultaneously vital and potentially hazardous. Among the positive aspects are modeling, developing a balance between skill and challenge, and enhancing the relationship between physical skills and positive self-attributions. Parents who themselves exercise set a model of full engagement with the world. Assisting children in learning at a level that provides challenge without overwhelming them can result in increased competence and enjoyment (Csikszentmihalyi, 1990). Conscious enhancement of self-esteem, physical competence, and psychological skills training can be a part of children's involvement in sport (Fine & Sachs, 1997).

As children move into youth sports, parental engagement and involvement shifts. Coaches take on a central role in children's development and sense of themselves. It is important to assess the parent-coach interaction, so that young athletes do not become triangulated in the process (Strean, 1995). Parental overinvolvement or overidentification is a particular risk, especially as children

> I run for about a half hour—leisurely pace—two to four times a week, first thing in the morning. Anyone in the family can come with me, as I will go at the slowest person's pace. This morning, my very out-of-shape 12-year-old son accompanied me and we had a good time together—walking whenever he needed. As a rule, the family golden retriever runs with us as well.
>
> **46-year-old male psychologist**

progress into higher levels of competition. Perhaps the best summary of optimal parental-child interaction—combining support, autonomy and role differentiation, modeling, and sport values—comes from a child advising parents about appropriate behavior in organized youth sport settings: "Shut up, sit down, watch the game quietly, and let your kid have fun" (Fine & Sachs, 1997, p.148).

PRACTITIONER RECOMMENDATIONS

Activity and play are primary ways in which children come to understand the world and themselves within the world. Therapeutic play and activity are means by which the child can express that sense of self and the therapist can understand the child.

To the extent that activity has direction and focus, the specific intent (e.g., the development of certain values) becomes important. Rather than assuming that these values will occur naturally with exercise or sport, the intent needs to be directed.

From the youngest age, children's activity is an opportunity for engagement that is gender neutral. Because many gendered assumptions are embedded within adults, it may take conscious effort and intention to shift such interactions.

Adolescents and Exercise

DISCUSSION

The majority of reported research concerning adolescents and exercise has focused on adolescents' involvement in sports. Gender-related research, described in chapter 15, supports the positive impact that sport or exercise can have on female adolescents' sense of self, self-esteem, and body image. As with younger children, use of activity as the medium in which psychotherapy can be conducted has a long tradition with adolescents.

A few studies have examined exercise as a stress-coping mechanism. For example, a study of 212 adolescent girls (mean age 13.8) enrolled in a private secondary school examined the function of exercise in buffering the effects of life stress (Brown & Siegel, 1988). A comparison of stress, illness, and exercise was made at two different time periods 8 months apart. Although there was a low rate of illness for all participants who experienced low levels of stress, those with high levels of stress had experienced significantly less illness if they also were high exercisers.

Brown and Siegel suggested that possible psychological mechanisms for the stress-coping effect included increased feelings of mastery and self-efficacy, with concomitant appraisal of life events as less stressful, or exercise as a respite from stressful life situations. Both of these explanations seem especially suited to adolescents, who are actively working on issues around self-efficacy and who may intensely experience life stressors as beyond their control.

Brown and Siegel noted that this was a homogeneous group with regard to socioeconomic status and race as well as gender, and their levels and types of physical activity may be different from the population at large, thus potentially limiting the generalizability of the findings. For example, the most common forms of exercise were aerobics, calisthenics, running, swimming, and tennis, rather than team sport activities.

Also looking at the buffering effect of activity on stress and adversity, Smith and Darling (1997) examined various extracurricular activities, including sports, among 8,000 high school students. Extracurricular activity involvement in general served as a buffer against adolescent substance use as well as the impact of family adversity. Additionally, sports involvement, specifically, served to buffer the impact of both family adversity and individual life stress.

> Concerned about her 13-year-old daughter's incipient eating disorder, Karen's mother contacted me, describing Karen's "nervous vomiting." And indeed, it was the adjective that was defining. Tall and rangy, Karen's childish face belied her cognitive poise and body's maturity. Earnestly, she said, "I tend to get nervous about a lot of things, and it goes to my stomach. I throw up." Caught between the sophisticated cliques of junior high school and her parents' recognition that she was still young though in a mature frame, Karen expressed these conflicts by avoiding social situations or finding her stomach unexpectedly heaving.
>
> An avid member of the local swim team, she had learned the rudiments of deep breathing in preparation for meets. She had never thought to generalize that calming method to other aspects of her life. With a bit of instruction to shore up her skill, and explanation of the function of anxiety and optimal levels of arousal (inverted U), Karen became curious and eager to tackle her discomfort.
>
> She began using deep breathing. Almost immediately, she became more aware of the frequency and extent of her nervousness. She also was responsive to relaxation imagery. Recalling a Caribbean vacation, she warmed to visualizing swimming with a dolphin. She easily adopted the kinesthetic anchor of the SCUBA thumb-to-forefinger circle to remind herself that she was emotionally okay. Pressing thumb and forefinger together became a cue to calm her breathing.
>
> Generalizing from her experience, Karen then brought these new skills to a peer mediation training session. She reinforced the teacher's training and taught her friends some new skills.

Given her initial presentation of anxiety in social situations, it was especially remarkable that she was able to demonstrate this new level of leadership without an upset stomach.

PRACTITIONER RECOMMENDATIONS

As with younger children, adolescents can be engaged therapeutically through physical activity. This can be especially useful if they are not particularly verbal or are not enthusiastic about working with a therapist. Additionally, since many adolescents experience concerns around self-esteem or body image, engagement in physical activity with them or discussion involving their sport or exercise involvement may address some of these issues as well.

Adolescents' sport involvement can be a means for connecting or elaborating on issues that may seem too emotionally charged or threatening if approached directly. As a nonverbal medium that can help regulate stress (endemic to adolescent experience), engagement in exercise can be particularly salubrious.

Exercise and the Elderly

DISCUSSION

As the general population cohort ages, increasing numbers of studies have demonstrated the beneficial effects of exercise among the elderly. This is truly an area that confirms the biopsychosocial nature of our being. In addition, the interactive effect, or virtuous rather than vicious, cycle, is demonstrated as well. In general, older adults with high self-efficacy for exercise, dietary fat, weight control, smoking, and alcohol consumption have better physical and mental health (Grembowski et al., 1993). In addition to the physical and social and emotional effects, exercise has been found to enhance cognitive functioning among the elderly in some studies (Heil & Henschen, 1996; Powell, 1974; Shephard, 1990; Stevenson & Topp, 1990). Fillingim and Blumenthal (1993) noted, however, variable results regarding improved cognitive functioning with this population, perhaps because of differences in duration of exercise training, experimental design, statistical analyses, participant characteristics, and selection of assessment instruments.

The Duke Aging and Exercise Study has examined many aspects of aging and exercise. One study focused especially on the effects of a

> I exercise regularly, swimming for 30 minutes 5 or 6 times a week and walking a mile 3 times a week. Ten years ago, I was still using the machines, but I decided that it was swimming which provided the best "feel good" experience.
>
> Exercise makes my life ever so much more enjoyable. I feel more optimistic. After my swim, I want to (and sometimes do) sing, "It's a Wonderful World." Even though she may have heard me say it a dozen times, when I leave the swim club, I sometimes say to the lady at the desk, "I feel 70 again."
>
> If I do not exercise, I feel slowed down, apathetic, sometimes even a little depressed.
>
> **86-year-old male psychologist**

long-term exercise program. Participants were 50 men and 51 women, ages 60–83, who were healthy, prior nonexercisers. They were randomly assigned among three groups: (a) aerobic exercise: 45 min of bicycle ergometry plus walking or mild jogging 3 times per week; (b) yoga 2 times per week, to provide comparable group support, attention, and social stimulation while controlling for effort (minimal cardiorespiratory impact); and (c) wait list controls for 16 weeks. Subsequently, all participants engaged in the aerobic exercise training regimen for 16 weeks. It is interesting to note that there was considerable demand among study participants to extend the training, and in response, the participants were given the option of participating in an additional 6 months of supervised aerobic exercise (14 months available in total). Fifty people, half of the participants, volunteered to continue.

At each level of aerobic exercise (i.e., 16 weeks or 14 months), there was significant and sustained increase in physical capacity while participants continued to exercise. Additionally, the men in the aerobic group obtained significant reduction in depression. Although other measures of psychological functioning did not show significant change, the participants perceived that they had changed. Blumenthal and colleagues (1991) commented that this perception may be important in and of itself, suggesting that certain exercise effects are more subtle than test instruments are capable of measuring.

A number of major research questions still exist concerning exercise and the elderly, such as longitudinal effects, that is, whether exercise throughout the life span can attenuate some of the cognitive declines associated with aging; whether exercise begun later in life can prevent further decline in functioning; and whether there are certain groups of elderly who would most benefit from exercise (Fillingim & Blumenthal, 1993).

For the past 5 years, psychologist Sara Wolff has run time-limited groups, entitled "Vital Aging: Transitions in Living and Aging" for women ranging in age from 68 to 92 and experiencing a variety of situational losses (Heitner, 1998). Along with reading and discussion, each group has included sessions conducted by a yoga instructor.

Barbara, 74, was referred by her physician for improved management of symptoms related to a hiatal hernia. She was able to understand that the more concerned she became about throat discomfort and problems in breathing, the more she experienced increased discomfort. Although her physician had conducted a variety of tests, all of which had proved negative, she was concerned that perhaps he still had not uncovered some obscure underlying cause.

Long widowed, Barbara enjoyed the combination of independence and connection available in sharing a two-family house with her son and his family. She seemed to pride herself on her health and independence and on not being perceived as old.

She was responsive to training in deep breathing and used the cue word "relax." Wondering if it might help to reinforce this increased calm, I recommended to her that she explore taking yoga classes. I also encouraged her to obtain more information about hiatal hernias, so that her health problems would not seem quite so mysterious to her.

Through telephone calls and fax, I also discussed this case at some length with her physician. He saw her as essentially quite healthy, but with increased complaining. He wondered if there were underlying issues that she was not identifying. (She remained resistant to any exploration of this in treatment.) I encouraged him to be as educative as he could be in appointments with her.

Barbara began learning yoga with a videotape, but continued to be anxious about her breathing. I commented that these problems sounded like they were a combination of reflux from the hernia plus anxiety. Confronting her, I suggested that she was in danger of becoming a hypochondriac. Hypochondriasis has been estimated to occur in 10–15% of older adults (APA, 1997). I taught her more elaborate (Jacobsonian) relaxation techniques, as well as a thought stopping process. I encouraged her, again, to discuss her physical concerns with her physician.

When seen for a final follow-up session a month later, she described feeling quite well. She noted that the reflux was markedly diminished and attributed it to decreased anxiety particularly through doing daily yoga on her own. She was about to start taking weekly classes.

Although she described a bit of family enmeshment, Barbara seemed ready to discontinue treatment, feeling confident that she was now able to handle things better on her own.

PRACTITIONER RECOMMENDATIONS

Increased research suggests that exercise in the elderly is helpful to the mind as well as the body. Yet it may not occur to the practitioner steeped in some of the same cultural assumptions as the elderly themselves to consider it as a treatment modality. Among clients in their 70s or 80s, there may be a sense of physical caution, a belief in retirement as physical stasis, and, especially among women, a lack of experience with physical activity as salubrious (Sara Wolf, personal communication, May 24, 1998). More than in the rest of the population, many elderly people may have beliefs and actions located in the precontemplation and contemplation stages of change. The stage of change model has been found to be equally applicable, with regard to exercise efficacy, to the elderly as to those who are younger (Gorely & Gordon, 1995). Thus, the practitioner may find it helpful to be familiar with and share various information regarding the mental as well as physical benefits of exercise.

Beyond the Game: 17
Athletes With Emotional Problems

Andrea, a college junior and Olympic hopeful, was referred to me by the college counseling center, after previous attempts at engaging her in psychotherapy, either through the counseling center or with a private therapist, had proved unsuccessful. In light of my sport psychology training, Andrea initially seemed willing to consider psychotherapy with me. And it was clear that her life was feeling out of control: Enmeshed in a long-term relationship with her considerably older coach-boyfriend, she was also ambivalently caught in issues with her divorced parents as well.

In our first session, we agreed to focus on both long- and short-term goal setting. Andrea easily shifted off focus, and seemed only marginally able to take in suggestions. Headed toward school break, she said she would call on return. She did not, and a call to her brought the response that she was swamped with work and training and would not continue in therapy at this time.

In many ways, Andrea is not an atypical student-athlete. In an early study, Pierce (1969) found college athletes less likely than other students to seek psychotherapy. Athletes apparently continue to underuse counseling services available to them (Cogan & Petrie, 1996a), perhaps because of a reluctance to admit weakness, desire for autonomy, teammates' social support, or fear that they will be perceived as deviant (Andersen, Denson, Brewer, & Van Raalte, 1994; Linder, Pillow, & Reno, 1989). Although the athlete seeking psychotherapy may be more comfortable working with a therapist knowledgeable about sport and respectful of its role in the athlete's life (Cogan, 1998; May, 1986), as with Andrea, this is no guarantee that a solid connection will be made.

Are athletes mentally healthier than the general population? Although Morgan (1985b) noted an "iceberg profile" on the Profile of Mood States, with "vigor" high and all other indices low, he also commented that because they are protected within the social structure, by the time athletes are diagnosed, those with problems may exhibit fairly severe psychopathology. Elsewhere, he observed, "The athlete who is in need of therapy exhausts all of his or her informal therapeutic options such as the team trainer, the team physician, the coaches, and his fellow athletes before he or she ends up in the psychiatrist's office" (The emotionally disturbed athlete, 1981, p. 71). Furthermore, out of a sense of community as well as protection of a financial asset, teams may accept psychotic behavior to protect the athlete.

There appear to be comparable rates of mental health problems of clinical significance among athletes and nonathletes (Mahoney & Suinn, 1986; Morgan, O'Connor, Sparling, & Pate, 1987) . Typical presenting problems include anxiety, depression, eating disorders, substance abuse, fears of success or failure, and relationship and motivational concerns (Mahoney & Suinn, 1986). Personality disorders, especially narcissistic personality disorder and antisocial personality disorder, have also been noted (Andersen et al., 1994).

In a roundtable discussion nearly 20 years ago (The emotionally disturbed athlete, 1981), four researcher-clinicians described a wide range of problems. The most frequent problem was depression, followed by substance abuse. Psychosomatic illnesses also were mentioned, triggered in part by athletes' reliance on their bodies and bodily functioning. Concern was expressed about characterological problems, especially among athletes in contact sports. "There are rewards and respect for the impulsive, aggressive person who tends to lash out or respond with hostility in a stressful situation" (p. 70). They also noted the challenge of finding the dividing line between appropriate rituals and superstition as compared with compulsive behavior that may indicate clinical significance. Further, one participant suggested, "These types of behavior are not emotional disturbances, because they are accepted by a subsociety" (p. 70). Not surprisingly for that time frame, only brief mention was made of eating disorders (anorexia nervosa). In that instance, the focus was placed on the need for medical, rather than psychological, management. Prognostically, early case finding was encouraged, so that when returning to play, the athlete would not have burned all his or her social bridges through earlier bizarre behavior.

> New York Mets pitcher Pete Harnisch's "mystery ailment" with symptoms of exhaustion, disrupted sleep and eating, anxiety, and emotional withdrawal was initially (mis)diagnosed as

nicotine withdrawal, thyroid condition, or Lyme disease. Ultimately, he was diagnosed as depressed. After Harnisch disclosed this diagnosis to the press, Allan Lans, M.D., director of the Mets' employee assistance program, commented, "It's understandable for an athlete to get a physical injury but not a mental injury. . . . If a player should get depressed, the sense is he should do it in the off-season . . . (Harnisch's) problem is ubiquitous; talking about it is rare." (Rich, 1997, p. A27)

Although the athlete with clinical problems in some ways is like any other patient or client presenting with clinical problems, the cultural context of the athlete's life must be taken into account. The nonathlete therapist can adopt a multicultural perspective, in which the arena of competitive sports is understood to represent a different culture (Mooney, 1993). In particular, the therapist needs to be open to difference and to understand the power and centrality of sports in the client's life and self-identification. This perspective can decrease a perception of sports participants as abnormal. In addition to an awareness of one's attitude toward athletes in general, the therapist needs to be clear about his or her attitudes toward specific subsets of athletes and issues, for example, women athletes, ethnicity, or sexual orientation (Cogan & Petrie, 1996b).

In this chapter I focus on four areas of concern, each of which may show increased prevalence among athletes as compared with the general population: substance abuse, eating disorders, sport performance phobic behavior, and sexual abuse. Substance abuse and eating disorders are problems that may be more likely to occur within athlete populations, in part as a function of the context of the athletic environment. Because it has been tied directly to competitive athletics, sport performance-related phobia is also described. And finally, for a number of reasons, treatment of athletes in relation to sexual abuse is also addressed. The athletic environment may be a contributing factor—and there is little published information on this important subject. Treatment of athletes suffering from emotional problems caused by overuse of exercise is described in chapter 18.

> Playing basketball feeds my competitive addiction. My day in the office focuses on cooperation but my Type A thrives on competitiveness. Playing basketball burns off excess irritations and keeps me in contact with young, vibrant, challenging people who make me appreciate health. It cleanses my body of the day's stresses and gives me a lift into the rest of the day's activities. It has brought with it the byproduct of camaraderie that only athletes seem to share: an appreciation of life. It is my art form and a way to express myself creatively (within the limits of my now diminishing skills). And, the number-one reason I play basketball: It is the most fun I can imagine and the best thing I share with my son.
>
> **51-year-old male psychologist**

Athletes and Substance Abuse

Alcohol and drug use within the athlete population occurs for a number of interrelated sociological and psychological reasons: It is a reflection of the use of substances within the general population; athletes may use substances to modulate emotions (up or down) related to the competitive environment and its pressures; and this type of use may be supported by the risk taking endemic to certain sports (Heil & Henschen, 1996).

Within professional sports, there is a direct connection between sports and alcohol use (Carr & Murphy, 1995). Advertisements for alcoholic beverages are central to televised sports events; brewing companies sponsor sports teams and events; recreational sports are social activities; and there is the implicit if not explicit isomorphism of sport, masculinity, and group alcohol use (Kunz, 1997). Further, "positive deviance" may positively sanction conformist behaviors that in other contexts would be viewed with concern (Coakley, 1997).

Within the sports culture, athletes encounter mixed messages and signals about the use of ergogenic or performance-enhancing drugs (Heil & Henschen, 1996). A variety of drugs serve different functions. Athletes may use anabolic steroids to increase muscular size and strength, drugs such as morphine for pain reduction, amphetamines to increase energy or arousal, beta-blockers to reduce arousal, or diuretics for weight control (Brewer & Petrie, 1996).

Specific gender differences in alcohol use have been noted within the general population, and there is no reason to think that athletes are different. In general, women begin both drinking and problem drinking later than men; develop alcohol dependence more rapidly than men; cite a specific stressor as the point of initiation of problem drinking; and, if alcohol use is problematic, describe themselves as feeling guilty, anxious, or depressed (Carr & Murphy, 1995).

Athletes and Eating Disorders

Along with a sports physician and the owner-coach of a gymnastics center, I participated in a radio program on adolescents and exercise. When the host asked about eating disorders, both of my colleagues showed an astounding lack of concern. "Oh," commented the gymnastics coach, "none of our students have eating disorders." Equally dismissive, the physician replied, "It's really typical for teenagers to have eating disorders. They grow out of it."

Frustrated with the inaccuracy of these comments, I did what I could to bring some sanity and information back to the discourse without totally shaming my colleagues. I complimented the gymnastics coach regarding participants in his particular program, but said that my understanding was that gymnastics was a high-risk sport for eating disorders. I also suggested that eating disorders can be or become complicated. Often, I explained, the trio of physician, nutritionist, and mental health practitioner is needed to assist in the resolution of these problems.

The truth about athletes and eating disorders is still not settled. We are moving from anecdote to evidence in relation to definition, predisposition, and prevalence. Intensive engagement in sports implies a powerful identification of oneself with one's body and its functioning. And yet there is a pull toward distortion. Athletes focus on all the aspects that may improve performance, including weight, diet, and appearance. "It is likely that most competitive athletes have been concerned with weight control at one time or another" (Swoap & Murphy, 1995, p. 307).

Compared with the general population, athletes are more concerned with body weight and use a wide array of pathological food behaviors (Brownell & Rodin, 1992). For many athletes, the primary means of weight control may appear invisible: exercise additional to one's sport participation.

A number of characteristics are common both to sports and to pathological weight control measures. Both anorexia and athletics involve hard work, perfectionism, a high need for achievement or superior performance, and the ability to withstand pain or discomfort (Thompson & Sherman, 1993). Sports participation involves competition, whether with oneself or with others.

The onset of eating disorders and competitive athletics typically occurs at the same developmental moment, adolescence. Further, eating disorders are most prevalent within certain demographics (White, middle- to upper-class adolescent girls), and these are exactly those girls who are most likely to engage in a number of competitive sports (Thompson & Sherman, 1993; Wilson & Eldredge, 1992).

In addition to the interaction of individual, familial, biological, and other sociocultural factors, sports participation itself may involve further pressures that move the individual toward an eating disorder (Thompson & Sherman, 1993; Thompson, 1996). The sport culture influences the individual through both the social surround and the sport itself. Davis et al. (1995) suggested that the mutual reinforcement of undereating and overexercising can be exacerbated for women within a sport or fitness environment that emphasizes obligatory commitment.

Sports that stress leanness, weight restriction, or attractiveness may heighten the likelihood of disregulated eating and weight preoccupation. "Thinness-demand" sports, such as long-distance running, are those in which leanness is related to performance. To compete in some sports, such as weight lifting, the athlete needs to meet certain weight classifications. Other sports, such as figure skating, include judging criteria based in part on current aesthetic definitions of physical attractiveness, thinness, and child-like qualities. These criteria may be directed with particular intensity toward girls (Brownell & Rodin, 1992; Petrie, 1996; Ryan, 1995; Swoap & Murphy, 1995; Wiese-Bjornstal, 1997; Wilson & Eldredge, 1992).

Although there is not yet clear enough information on the interaction between eating disorders and elite levels of competition, especially in thinness-demand sports, logic and anecdotal evidence would suggest yet further pressures toward weight control that may become pathological. *Little Girls in Pretty Boxes: The Making and Breaking of Elite Gymnasts and Figure Skaters* (Ryan, 1995), details the underside of elite sports, the pressures of stardom, money, perfectionism, coach and parental pressures concentrated on body- and identity-insecure adolescent girls. Ryan described, for example, the struggles of Kristie Phillips, a gymnast groomed for the Olympics from age 4 to 16. Through diuretics and laxatives, she lost 10 pounds in 3 weeks—and lost strength and energy as well. When she did not qualify for the Seoul Olympics, her despair was profound. She concluded, "I'm never going to make it in life because I'm fat" (Ryan, 1995, p. 116). She subsequently embarked on years of bulimic behavior.

In part because of measurement issues, the comparative prevalence of diagnosable eating disorders among athletes and nonathletes is not clear. In a large sample of female collegiate gymnasts, Petrie and Stoever (1993) found a 4% prevalence rate of bulimia nervosa, somewhat lower than other estimates. There may, however, be increased pathogenic weight control behaviors—themselves often considered potential precursors to eating disorders. Student athletes surveyed by Petrie and Stoever, for example, reported exercising excessively to lose weight (57%), fasting or going on a strict diet (28%), and vomiting (6%).

When one compares female athletes (lean sport and nonlean sport) with female nonathletes, the female athletes in general express more positive feelings of worth and effectiveness, as well as satisfaction with body shape, as measured by the Eating Disorders Inventory. In general, male athletes and nonathletes focus more on strength and muscle mass than weight preoccupation per se (Petrie, 1996).

> Having always enjoyed wrestling, on returning to college 28-year-old Mark made the wrestling team but then experienced considerable doubt and ambivalence about his functioning on

the team. He commented, "I want to be good enough to compete. I feel like I'm insulting this sport I love. I set unrealistic goals for myself and then quit."

Therapy focused on helping Mark develop and maintain reasonable goals for himself, taking into account a long history of low self-confidence and self-esteem. As he began creating a system for physical training, it became clear that he had no overall sense of his own capabilities. His life involved impulsive decision making. Consistent with this was his intention to drop either 11 or 19 pounds within a short period of time so as to qualify for wrestling competition at a certain weight class. He would combine fasting with sweating off the pounds.

This type of disregulated eating, or "transient abnormal eating behavior" (Wilson & Eldredge, 1992, p. 123), can be normative within the sport subculture. Attempting to qualify at certain classes of weight, many wrestlers engage in this kind of behavior. Abnormal weight control for an instrumental purpose, it is not strictly an eating disorder. Without body distortion and weight preoccupation, this behavior does not have attached to it the kind of self-perpetuating psychophysiological baggage of an eating disorder. Generally, the effects are not markedly detrimental. Further, as a man, Mark was not carrying the weight messages of the culture. Still, the pathogenic potential of disregulated eating should not be ignored.

Mark was able to recognize that his intended weight loss method might be counterproductive: Although he might lose the weight, an additional result could be dehydration and decreased competitive prowess. He was able to take a slightly longer term view, recognizing that an increase in aerobic exercise and food moderation could result in goal attainment within a few weeks rather than a few days, along with a greater sense of accomplishment and control.

Athletes' attitudes concerning the interaction of eating, weight, weight management, and performance are often influenced by key participants in their lives. The roles of coaches, parents, and peers all can be significant. Pressure from the central figure in the athlete's life, the coach, can be especially intense and overdetermined. Parents' own identity and money may ride on the young athlete's performance. Peer culture, central to all adolescents, can be especially influential for a team- or sport-identified youngster.

Given the feminine attunement to social perceptions of others, and the degree of sensitization that females in our culture experience in relation to issues of food or weight, these attitudes and the way that they are conveyed can be crucially important for girls and women. In a survey of high school coaches, Griffin and Harris (1996) found a number of troubling attitudes and beliefs about weight. Coaches indicated negative feelings about overweight people. Male coaches blamed obesity on character (laziness) rather than behavior (eating the wrong foods; history of crash diets); viewed weight as highly important in their sport; thought that female athletes needed to lose weight and male athletes needed to gain weight; used appearance as the primary means of judging whether athletes needed to lose or gain weight; recommended a variety of weight loss techniques; and referred their athletes to physicians, nutritionists, and trainers (but not psychotherapists).

> Shannon, a 15-year-old, was referred by her guidance counselor because of concerns that she might have an incipient eating disorder. Family and friends noted picky eating and weight obsession. Her menses also were disrupted, and she exhibited a driven, perfectionistic personality. Shannon, an avid runner, expressed willingness to work with me because of my involvement in sport psychology.
>
> We started our work near the end of the school year, and once school ended, much of the tension and food and weight preoccupation she had been experiencing receded. Although she enjoyed a variety of summer activities, she also wanted to follow a training schedule in order to be prepared for the fall cross-country running season. I encouraged her to check with her coach. When she did, he not only gave her a training schedule but also counseled her to gain about 10 pounds in order to run better. Encouraged by this advice, and with the support of a nutritionist to whom I had also referred her, Shannon began to feel more comfortable paying attention to her actual sensations of hunger. She began to think about other arenas in which to express her competitiveness.
>
> Thoroughly impressed with the coach's intervention, I checked with Shannon, and with her very willing permission, I called the coach to let him know how pivotal his recommendation was to Shannon's healthy development.

Athletes and Phobic Behavior

Phobias may be frequent in athletes at all levels of sport (The emotionally disturbed athlete, 1981). Silva (1994) has described "sport performance phobias" as sharing characteristics with simple, social, and agoraphobia, as well as with music performance anxiety. He suggests that these phobias have specific characteristics: There is always an acute onset or episodic event; and the phobia is specific, related to only one aspect of the athlete's entire performance which prior to that point has been (a) routine or (b) central to the athlete's positional function. These two salient characteristics seemed to determine an athlete's experience of internal threat. "All athletes reported an immense sense of loss of physical control, physical and psychological weakness and disorientation" (p. 104). Additionally, they experienced guilt about letting down the team, significant others, and themselves. They described an intense anticipation of personal embarrassment, marked anticipatory anxiety and desire to not perform the behavior in question, and a behavior-specific decrease in confidence. The athletes felt a need to compensate for this area of poor performance, and experienced a strong desire to leave the playing field during competition. Since this type of phobia often occurred during a playing season, Silva recommended that the consultant should implement the intervention as rapidly and efficiently as possible (i.e., through increased intensity, such as daily meetings). Prompt treatment may preclude further accumulated negative experiences.

Athletes and Sexual Abuse

> Stephanie, age 29, sought therapy for depression that derived in part from a history of marked emotional and physical parental neglect. She experienced pervasive discomfort with emotional and physical intimacy. In addition to familial neglect, this discomfort appeared directly related to her history as a gymnast: She recalled, with shame, the frequent, continual stare and touch of her gymnastics coach as she and her sisters practiced their routines throughout their childhood.

DISCUSSION

Almost no information is available concerning the prevalence of sexual abuse among those within the athlete community. As with other issues mentioned in this chapter, there is no reason to believe that rates of sexual abuse among athletes are not similar to the general population (Cogan & Petrie, 1996a). Taking into account not only a history of familial or extrafamilial abuse but also contemporaneous sexual exploitation (e.g., by coaches), it is possible that rates may in fact be higher. Athletes may be at increased risk in some instances, given a combination of the sexism found in organized sports; a focus on the physical self; close-fitting clothing; marked power differentials; positively sanctioned touching (for instruction or to indicate camaraderie); the prevalence of male coaches; and the intense emotional intimacy of the sport environment. Sport culture, especially at high levels of certain sports, often encourages marked, almost familial, intimacy between player and coach. Furthermore, coaches have available to them a number of types of power: reward power, coercive power, legitimate power, expert power, and charismatic or referent power (Brackenridge, 1994).

The most extensive writing on this subject is a chapter, "My coach says he loves me," in sports investigative reporter Nelson's *The Stronger Women Get, the More Men Love Football* (1994). Finding parallels between coaches and other men in authority, Nelson points to the potential for abuse of power and trust in sports. "While a coach may with one hand reach to help a woman free herself of sexist constraints through athletic achievement, he may with the other hand seduce her, thus effectively trapping her in a sexualized, dependent position" (p. 163). The negative sanctions that exist for other people in comparable positions of authority, (e.g., ethics codes in psychotherapist organizations) are lacking in many sports, and many coaches are averse to such sanctions. Because athletics is an important revenue base for a school, persons in authority also may be reluctant to take action if abuse is suspected. If the relationship between athlete and coach becomes legitimized through dating or marriage, it is generally accepted, even though, as with Andrea, mentioned at the beginning of this chapter, there may be a wide discrepancy in age and power in the relationship.

"'What about the lesbians?' Bring up the topic of coach-athlete sex and inevitably, men mention lesbians" (Nelson, 1994, p. 188). There are instances of women coaches inappropriately involved with their student-athletes, yet there is so much homonegativity within sports that it becomes difficult to distinguish whether this is a genuine concern about abuse or another attempt to distort women's roles and protect those of men in sports. Again, there is no information on the frequency of such abuse. Even if one were to guess that there were twice as many lesbian abuse experiences as in the nonathlete population, that would still bring the ratio of male abusers to female abusers to approximately 92:8.

Since men are by far more likely to be perpetrators, it is interesting that it is only within the past few years that instances have become public of male coaches who have sexually abused boys. Eight years after having been abused, then-Boston Bruins player Sheldon Kennedy brought a suit against his junior hockey coach, Graham James.

> The coach is so respected. Your parents send you away and say, "Do what he says." At that age, you listen. . . . He was really a nice guy. . . . He didn't have to scare you, although he had a shotgun when he was laying in bed. (A supporting cast, June 19, 1997)

Psychotherapy for people who have been sexually abused or exploited has undergone considerable support, controversy, and attack in the past number of years (Courtois, 1988; Herman, 1992; Pope &

Brown, 1996). Conducting psychotherapy with an athlete with abuse issues involves knowledge both of the sport culture and of treatment for sexual abuse resolution.

PRACTITIONER RECOMMENDATIONS

This book is directed to psychotherapists who may not have formal training in or knowledge about the field of sport psychology. At the same time, when working with athletes, the more the therapist knows about athletes, the athlete culture, and the specific sport, the stronger the likelihood that a therapeutic bond may develop. At the very least, it is important for therapists to have a respectful interest in the world and context in which the client operates.

Recently, Gould and Damarjian (1998) and Van Raalte (1998) offered advice to practitioners working with athletes in competitive or elite sport environments. Athletes, they suggested, are most responsive when practitioners working with them understand the central role of sport in their lives, appreciate their time constraints, use and understand correct sport terminology, have sport specific knowledge, and are practical.

Athletes may dismissively view nonathletes as "civilians," unfamiliar with the world of sport (Cogan, 1998). Along with recognizing the athlete's culture, the therapist also may have the task of acculturating the athlete to the non-sport-specific, therapeutic expertise that the therapist has to offer.

Athletes come to therapy with a number of strengths and capabilities. They are used to having a strong sense of discipline in their activities. Additionally, they are accustomed to responding to instruction, to practicing new skills, and to focusing internally on changes, albeit somatic rather than psychic changes. All of these attributes suggest that when the therapist makes suggestions or gives homework assignments—particularly if they are written out—the level of compliance may be considerably higher than when one makes suggestions to other, less focused, therapy clients.

If the athlete is experiencing both clinical and performance enhancement issues, collaboration with another practitioner may allow the client to receive optimal service (Andersen et al., 1994; Brodsky & Ravizza, 1985; Yambor & Connelly, 1991). This teamwork may be initiated either by the psychotherapist or by the psychological skills trainer. The collaboration can be either conjoint, or, if effective communication between helping professionals is maintained, separate and simultaneous.

IV | CAVEATS AND BOUNDARIES

When Bad Things Happen to Good Sports:

The Consequences of Overuse

18

Having extolled the virtues of exercise, it is also important to acknowledge ways in which it can be overdone. For the nonathlete everyday exerciser, the likelihood of overuse is fairly slight, more in the nature of "man bites dog"—rare, although possible. However, since this concern is raised at times, and since overuse does occur, and furthermore, since therapists can be helpful in resolving this problem, it is useful to understand this issue. In this chapter I focus on a number of interrelated concerns with regard to people who exercise regularly—whether they are weekend warriors, committed exercisers, collegiate athletes, or professional athletes. Various costs—to the mind as well as the body— are described; experimental studies on exercise deprivation are summarized; theoretical models of exercise overuse are presented; and detailed case examples illustrate the interaction of psychosocial history, current stressors, and exercise injury.

The Psychophysiological and Psychosocial Costs

As Dave Barry would say, this is a true story:

> I am at the New York City Marathon, doing brief mental skills training interventions as a member of the Psyching Team. A worried looking man

approaches me to ask whether I think he should run. He explains that on the previous day he was given an EKG and obtained "equivocal" results. His physician expressed some concern to him. The physician also mentioned the words Jim Fixx—the runner and popularizer of running who died of a heart attack while running—to the man's wife. I ask the man some questions about his health and risk factors. He appears immovably indecisive. Finally, concerned that I am getting nowhere and may be medically in over my head, I introduce him to Harold Selman, M.D., the psychiatrist who co-leads the Psyching Team. He asks similar questions and receives correspondingly inconclusive replies. Harold assures the man a place in the race the following year if he decides not to run this year. Still, nothing settled. Finally Harold pulls out the big card: "Which is more important," he asks, "your life or this race?" At this, the man suddenly draws himself up, all doubt resolved. With conviction, he states, "I'll run."

The next day I carefully check the *New York Times*. There are no reports of death on the race course.

Do people who exercise sometimes get weird about their exercise? Yes. Is that weirdness sometimes overdetermined? Of course. Depending on the person, exercising too much may involve some combination of inappropriate goals, invincibility, drivenness, compensation, displacement, stress management, psychophysiological responsiveness, as well as a response to others' demands or expectations. The extreme situation described in the vignette above is a rationale used by some to justify not exercising at all.

In our quintessentially American faith that more is better, we sometimes are caught in a dangerous trap. Exercise in moderation can indeed lead to improved self-concept, mastery, self-efficacy, self-sufficiency, body image, and cognitive processing, yet too much exercise can result in negative effects. Whether overtraining to meet performance goals (Raglin, 1993) or attempting to control weight—or life—through compulsive or obligatory exercise (Yates, 1991), people who exercise more than their bodies can tolerate are at increased risk of sustaining specific as well as training stress injuries. Physiological signs include sleep disturbance, increased illness and injury, chronic muscle soreness, and elevated resting heart rate and blood pressure. Psychosocial symptoms, such as fatigue, problems with concentration, apathy, anger, irritability, depression, and impaired social relations, may be even more apparent. Sport performance deteriorates. In a futile attempt to improve performance, the athlete may then exacerbate the problem by increasing training (Henschen, 1993; McCann, 1995; Raglin, 1993). Although the major prescription for chronic training stress is a decrease in activity, clients who exercise intensively may be markedly resistant to such a suggestion.

The therapist's diagnostic and therapeutic tasks are many: to understand the antecedents, to recognize the internal and external forces maintaining the person's current situation, and, ultimately, to assist the person in developing a more balanced life. At the same time, it is critically important to take into account the client's own context and values, so as not to overpathologize the situation. Especially for the therapist or consultant without involvement in physical activity or a background in sports, it may be valuable to use a multicultural perspective to fully appreciate athletic commitment (Mooney, 1993). An athlete's coach, for example, may be systematically increasing the training load, and improved performance and maintenance of a college scholarship may depend on complying with training expectations.

Exercise Degradation

Jason, 47, tense and restless, was referred by the local psychologists' referral service. His initial complaint was that he was "addicted to exercise." A man without relationships ("I haven't had any relationships for a long time—I'd drive someone crazy") and chronically unemployed because of frequent (exercise-related) injury, he lived at home with his parents. He described an "agitated depression" that occurred about 10 years previously concurrent with other behavioral changes, including an increase in smoking, alcohol consumption, and very intense working out with weights. He also was sleepless. He was hospitalized for 3 weeks. Experiencing the medications (Valium and Sinequan) to be irritants, he discontinued them.

He reported some prior attempts at psychotherapy. Currently, he said he "would like to be in control, to be able to back off [exercise] when I get sore." Instead, he was finding himself lifting heavier weights more frequently. "It just builds up again until I get injured."

Jason described himself as basically insecure, moody, and grouchy. He also said that he couldn't sit still and, indeed, his level of agitation during the interview conveyed a palpable tension.

He was neither an especially articulate nor insightful informant, and the prospect for reflective, exploratory psychotherapy seemed unlikely. Differential diagnostic possibilities included bipolar disorder, schizotypal personality disorder, obsessive–compulsive disorder, and attention deficit hyperactivity disorder (ADHD), the latter being one about which Jason expressed some curiosity as well. The immediate issue involved helping him redirect his method of tension management in order for it be less physically and mentally debilitating.

My strategy was twofold: gear him toward more somatically soothing exercise, so that exercise could have its intended effect without negative consequences, and develop a clearer diagnostic understanding.

Although he reported some experience with self-hypnosis, I taught him deep breathing in great detail, focusing especially on triangle and square breathing. I recommended that he practice the breathing at least 4 times a day and described it as similar to medication—except with no negative side effects. On a 1–10 scale, I explained, with deep breathing he could self-monitor the level of bodily stress he was experiencing, striving to keep it below a 7.

I encouraged Jason to find out about available yoga classes and gave him a few phone numbers to get more detailed information. Such activity could provide a systematic means of exercise that would not be harmful and could also give him an opportunity for some social interaction. And, since he lived at home, I suggested that he do some fact finding about his early development, as a first step toward understanding whether ADHD was implicated in his problems. I gave him a series of questions about his developmental history that he could ask his parents.

Scheduled to come in for an appointment 2 weeks later, Jason called about 10 days later to cancel the appointment. He felt that he had received the help that he had needed. Much to his surprise, the breathing exercises were helping a lot; he was checking into yoga classes; and he was reconsidering the question of medication. I had no further contact with him.

The notion that exercise leads one to feel good and the popular use of the terms "endorphins" or "runner's high" can leave us believing that exercise produces specific positive chemical changes. Scientific proof has not yet caught up with this popular perspective, however. The biochemistry and physiology of exercise and mood are much more complicated than at first appears. At best, the relationship may not be entirely linear, or the function of one specific factor. Consider, for example:

- Mood change can occur even after exercise of insufficient intensity to elicit significant endorphin production;
- A clear dose-response relationship between acute exercise intensity and positive mood change has not yet been established;
- In fact, at higher FIT (high intensity chronic training) there is a sharp decrement in mood (Hoffman, 1997; Raglin, 1997).

A few experimental studies have attempted to examine the connection between exercise and mood. The underlying premise of these studies has been that one way to prove the causal link between exercise and improved mood states is to test the polar opposite of this proposition: to see if mood deteriorates with exercise deprivation. It has been notoriously challenging to conduct such experiments, since habitual exercisers are rarely willing to discontinue exercise (Sachs, 1981). Research, often methodologically flawed, has indicated experimental effects. However, it has been difficult to tease out the degree to which these effects are psychological as compared with physiological.

> When I'm exercising, my thinking is less task-oriented, less "tight," and much more meditative and sensory-involved. A free and released thinking. It is often a time of simply coming to terms with feelings and situations. But this does not mean it is not focused—the mind-body connection is stronger. I think and image my goals and they happen. It's very hypnotic or zen-like when things are going well. Even on days when it is harder to relax and get into the rhythm of the workout, I usually find at the end, when I stop or return to work, that I experienced some meditative level that clearly nourished me. I find that I meet frustration in my exercise routinely only when I try to push to do an external goal rather than the level of activity that feels right at that moment.
>
> **34-year-old female social worker**

Three recent studies have noted marked psychological and physiological changes with exercise deprivation. In one, 40 male volunteers were recruited after a marathon and randomly assigned to either 2 weeks of running deprivation or (exercise) control (Morris, Steinberg, Sykes, & Salmon, 1990). Somatic and subjective symptoms (problems with sleep, ability to cope) were noticeable in the first week. By the second week of deprivation there were appreciable increases in anxiety and depression. Once the deprived group resumed running, the groups no longer differed. Using an experience sampling method over 35 days, Gauvin and Szabo (1992) randomly assigned male and female college students, highly committed to exercise, to either an exercise deprivation (refrain from exercising Days 15–21) or a control condition. The experimental participants reported more physical symptoms (e.g., headaches, muscle tension) than at baseline and in comparison with the control group during and following the week of exercise withdrawal, but no increase in mood disturbance. Mondin and colleagues (1996) measured the levels of anxiety and depression in 10 habitual exercisers. These people (male and female, with a mean age of 27 years, who typically exercised a minimum of 45 min a day, 6 or more days a week), took the State–Trait Anxiety Inventory (STAI), Profile of Mood States (POMS), and Depression Adjective Checklist daily for 5 days. They exercised on the first and last day, but refrained during the middle three days. There was a significant increase on all measures of distress during the exercise deprivation phase.

Models of Overuse: Staleness, Burnout, and Addiction

To explain the phenomenon of exercise degradation, researchers have extrapolated from other models. Various disagreements have arisen around conceptualization and semantics in this process. In a manner somewhat reminiscent of Lewis Carroll, at times the same words are used to mean different things, and in other instances, different words mean the same thing. Some concepts are useful more for their metaphorical than literal value. Some may translate directly from other domains, whereas others may be sport-specific (Raglin, 1993). To avoid confusion or misinterpretation, it is helpful to understand various terms, their derivation and their meaning.

Three overlapping models of the overuse of exercise are intertwined: stress models, burnout, and addiction or medical models. Selye's stress theory describes a three-stage physiological response to stressors that continue beyond an optimal level: alarm, resistance, and exhaustion (Selye, 1956). As applied in sport psychology, psychophysiological deterioration occurs as the body gradually becomes unable to cope with chronic training stress. In the stress model, "overtraining" refers to a deliberate strategy by which athletes are exposed to an ever-increasing intensity of training, designed to maximize performance, especially in endurance sports. Although intended to help the athlete peak at the time of a certain event, this performance demand can be costly, both physiologically and psychologically (Berger & Owen, 1992b; Morgan et al., 1988). In this model, the process of adding stressors—overtraining—can be distinguished from the potentially negative outcome of performance decrement—staleness.

The term *burnout,* developed initially by Freudenberger (1977), and elaborated by Maslach (1982), is familiar to most therapists as well as the lay public. Burnout characteristics include: (a) emotional and physical exhaustion, including a loss of concern, energy, interest, and trust; (b) depersonalization, a negative change in an individual's response to others, loss of fellow feeling, and cynicism; and (c) a sense of low personal accomplishment: low self-esteem, feelings of failure, and depression.

Smith (1986) was the first to adapt burnout theory to sport. Subsequently, combining elements of both stress theory and burnout, Silva (1990) argued persuasively for a continuum model, as compared with an all-or-none perspective. The imposition of training stress, which he referred to as overload, can result in positive or negative adaptation to that stress. Over time, and with the continued imposition of training stress, detraining effects emerge, such that there is a gradual deterioration from staleness to overtraining to burnout.

Arguing against the burnout model, Raglin (1993) suggested that staleness (his term for the end state) is unique to sport. The characteristic burnout element of loss of interest or motivation is not present, and the mood disturbance is directly related to training load.

The third explanation, addiction, uses a pathology model. Sometimes referred to as exercise compulsion or dependence, more commonly it is described as exercise addiction or negative addiction. The addiction analogy derives particularly from William Glasser's *Positive Addiction* (1976). Glasser suggested that certain activities, such as running and meditation, could help provide increased psychological health and life satisfaction for people. These are positive habits to which people may become addicted. People speak of becoming hooked on exercise, or needing their fix for the day. Some people who exercise regularly become habituated, consequently needing more exercise to experience the same effects (Morgan, 1985b). Further, if one does not engage in the addictive activity, there may be a number of negative consequences. Both somatic and psychological symptoms of withdrawal may be experienced, such as anxiety, restlessness, guilt, irritability, tension, frustration, depression, sleep problems, digestive tract difficulties, and muscle tension (Sachs, 1981; Williams & Roepke, 1993). By way of corroborative illustration, Sachs noted that it was difficult to investigate the process by which addiction develops, since potential participants were unwilling to stop running long enough for their responses to be studied.

The idea of positive and negative addiction has tremendous intuitive appeal. Add to that the physiological component of the "feel good" phenomenon when one is exercising, and, conversely, irritability and depression when one does not exercise, and the psychophysiological interconnection becomes at least metaphorically transparent.

The therapist who appreciates the perspectives provided by these three models can learn to work flexibly to comprehend nuance and convey information. When a coach or athlete describes overtraining, the therapist can sort out whether this refers to intentional overload training or is a negative consequence of overuse. Similarly, it would be important to clarify whether staleness refers to marginal difficulty or utter depletion. Depending on the client, the face validity of burnout or addiction may communicate more effectively than some of the more technical terms.

Remediation

Regardless of terminology, reports of athletes in various sports and at different levels of competitiveness suggest that three out of four will experience at least some level of psychophysiological distress, and as many as half or more experience the most severe levels of distress related to overuse of exercise (Raglin, 1993; Silva, 1990). Thus, this phenomenon appears quite frequently in highly trained individuals for whom physical activity has a marked degree of salience.

> George, a 30-year-old triathlete, was referred for psychotherapy by his orthopedic surgeon. He was not cooperating with the physician's treatment recommendations for complete rest to resolve tendinitis, an inflammation of the tendons in his legs. The orthopedist had prescribed a 4–6 week moratorium on exercise, and George found this intolerable. He had tried an occasional day off from working out, but as soon as the pain eased, he resumed his routine.
>
> George described himself as currently short-tempered, overwhelmed at work, gloomy, tired, and enervated. A gangly, adolescent-looking man, George was emotionally immature as well. He had few friends, no history of dating, and a highly stressful and unsatisfying job. Triathlon competitions provided a major focus for his life and structure to his self-definition.
>
> Evaluation and treatment of George involved attention to his belief system, the effects of his early history, and his characteristic defenses, resistance, and strength. It also was important to educate him concerning training degradation, so that he could come to appreciate the fact that his depression was actively related to the physiological stress he was placing on his body.
>
> During the first session, I focused on the presenting problem: George's unwillingness to stop exercising long enough to heal. At one level, he recognized the validity and importance of his physician's recommendation. And yet the thought of even a week's respite was unimaginable to him.
>
> To underscore the conflicting views he held, we developed a list of the beliefs that were preventing George from resting, as well as some rational responses he might use to challenge those assumptions. For example, when he worried about losing conditioning after a day or two, he could remind himself: "I'd maintain enough, and it would come back, especially if I continue with swimming and Nautilus." Whereas his first thought was, "If I don't do this physical activity or compete, it feels like someone's pulled my legs out from under me," he recognized the need to attend to other sources of self-esteem. He had been labeling himself a failure and yet acknowledged, "Other athletes have to take time off too—and they don't like it either."
>
> Over the next few sessions, more of George's history and its relevance to his current dilemma emerged. He had grown up the only child of an alcoholic mother and physically abusive

stepfather. George's response to family tension during childhood had been activity. He had attempted to stave off his mother's negative moods and his stepfather's punishment by being studious and cooperative, leaving the house quickly, often, and for as long as possible. He would wander outside for hours, dreading the return home.

The thought of discontinuing physical activity allowed George to understand the emotional connection between his childhood experience and his anxiety. For the first time, he spoke of some of the pain of his childhood, and, despite his introversion, found social, intellectual, and emotional solace in a short-term group for adult children of alcoholics to which I referred him. He was responsive to relaxation training and began broadening his repertoire of enjoyed activities and alternative coping resources.

George began pacing himself more reasonably at work. He focused increasingly on the present moment, recognizing that his life was no longer fraught with psychic and physical danger that needed to be warded off through compulsive physical activity. As he understood more about his characteristic approach to stress, George began to develop perspective on his triathlon training. He drew a graph of his prior racing season, rating three factors on a 1–10 scale: the amount of work stress he had been experiencing at the time, his intensity of training, and his actual race performance. (Like many competitive athletes, he had no difficulty recalling race events, conditions, and experiences.) From this graph, George could immediately see two significant facts he had been emotionally unable to grasp. More training did not necessarily result in improved race performance. Further, his always-stressful job became seasonally more challenging exactly at peak racing time.

This graph proved a turning point for George's life planning: He began designing a more reasonable and pleasurable approach to the next racing season, choosing 2-event, rather than 3-event, races. Despite some job adjustments, he recognized that he was chronically unhappy in that work setting. After reflection and discussion, he quit his current job, opting to try his hand at work that he enjoyed.

With regard to the precipitant for psychotherapy, George ultimately was able to tolerate 2 weeks without running or bicycling, although he continued to swim the entire time. The tendinitis healed. In the process, George learned to systematize his training, including giving his body both planned and fortuitous respite.

This client's experience offers a vivid example of the insidious effects of overuse on the psyche as well as on the body. The ability to moderate exercise is often much more complex than just saying no. Diagnostically, one could understand George from a variety of perspectives: psychophysiology, psychodynamics, and metacognitions. And he was responsive to a variety of therapeutic techniques. George's case also provides an opportunity to recognize the limits of individual psychotherapy, as well as the importance of adjunctive treatments. George was able to profit from his group experiences. Further, it seemed evident that his prior approach to athletic training was haphazard and probably contributed to his injury. Rather than design a training schedule for him, I encouraged him to read and consult with a fitness trainer or coach to create a more systematic method for the upcoming training season. He was thus able to further empower himself.

Practitioner Recommendations

At what point does athletic training move from pressured to taxing? When does exercise shift from enjoyable to driven? Although this transition may be idiosyncratic, it may well be internally consistent for the individual. This slippery slope involves a combination of exercise history, current physiological demand, and other psychosocial pressures and stressors. The task of the therapist may be to help the exercising person recognize his or her own particular warning signs. Despite the availability of fine-tuned physiological measurement, for therapists there is something reassuring and validating about the fact that psychological signs are often more accurate predictors than physiological indicators (Morgan et al., 1988).

The sport psychology literature suggests a number of strategies for slowing the development of negative stress response or recovering from it (Fender, 1989; Henschen, 1998; McCann, 1995; Sachs, 1981). The athlete can schedule some off-periods during which he or she does not exercise at all, although, as I mentioned, it is widely recognized that this method is difficult to implement. Cross-training, involving other sports that use different muscles, may be more appealing. Weight training, for example, may become a substitute for running a few days per week, thus increasing upper body strength while giving the legs a rest. Participating in other competitive activities can maintain the fighting edge without compromising the body. Engaging in noncompetitive, nonstressful social team activities, likewise, can enhance the sense of peer connection without bodily strain.

One of the dynamics involved in overuse is the attempt to maintain control. The person who is able to make choices about the training schedule may feel an increased sense of being in control. Coping strategies can be discussed in advance to deal with anticipated negative thoughts and feelings that may be a consequence of decreased physical activity. A logbook or journal can be useful for a variety of reasons: The client can record some of those cognitions and affects. Additionally, the journal allows one to track and ultimately predict periods of high training stress. Planning mental practice periods, in which one uses mental imagery of the sport, can serve to break up the monotony of practice, allow the body to recuperate physically, and help the client recognize the utility of mental methods. For those involved in competitive sports, learning how to handle postcompetition tension also can serve a preventative function, since some postcompetition reactions may relate to training stress.

Being Fit:
Ethical Issues Relevant to Exercise and Therapy

19

The various psychotherapy professions have a well-established history of codifying ethical principles (e.g., APA, 1992). Some 45 years ago, for example, as psychology newly engaged in psychotherapy practice on a large scale, APA developed its first ethics code. Currently that code is in the process of its eighth revision.

Each therapist must be guided by her or his relevant professional code. The practitioner interested in exercise in therapy also will find it instructive to be aware of a separate document specifically designed to address exercise and sport psychologists, the Ethical Principles and Standards of the Association for the Advancement of Applied Sport Psychology (Meyers, 1995). Although drawing heavily from APA's Ethical Principles and Code of Conduct, AAASP's document is designed to address some of the issues specific to this emerging field. It takes into account the interdisciplinary training, role, and settings of those engaged in exercise and sport psychology (Whelan, Meyers, & Elkin, 1996). Although these principles and codes are designed specifically for sport psychologists, therapists incorporating exercise in their practice would do well to understand and use them as appropriate. (For a detailed discussion of the AAASP Principles and Standards, as well as an excellent summary of philosophies of ethics undergirding the professions of psychology and sport psychology, the interested reader is encouraged to review Whelan, Meyers, & Elkin, 1996.)

A Comparison of Documents

APA's Ethical Principles and Code and AAASP's Principles and Standards are similar in their overall structure and content. Each contains an introductory explanation, a guiding preamble, and a set of six principles, followed by a series of enforceable rules or standards of ethical conduct. Whereas APA has 102 standards clustered into 8 sections, AAASP has 25 such standards. Certain sections of the APA standards, such as forensic activities, are not included within the AAASP standards, since they are generally irrelevant to the role requirements of applied sport psychology.

Within the AAASP document, the following differences provide a notable contrast to those of the APA: an absence of restriction on sexual activity with former clients; more exacting prohibition against barter; less focus on social responsibility; and less stringent prohibition of testimonials, but greater sensitivity to ways in which athlete visibility may be especially challenging to the sport psychologist. These differences appear to reflect the interdisciplinary training and practice focus in an emerging profession, as well as the role complexity of the practicing sport psychologist.

Therapists are encouraged to comply with the most stringent expectations of their profession. Issues that may be especially salient to therapists' work with clients in regard to exercise are those with regard to competence, confidentiality, boundaries, and diagnosis.

Competence

The word *competence* derives from the Latin and, appropriate to the focus of this book, means "being fit." Competence underlies the medical injunction to "do no harm" and moves beyond proscription to capacity and proficiency.

Rather than being a unitary concept, competence comprises a number of facets. Competence to do what? In assessing one's own training, one's skills, and one's presentation to the public, it is useful for the practitioner to ask not only, "What am I competent at?" but also "What am I not competent at?" Further, thinking proactively, it is important to assess: "How do I want to handle areas in which I am not competent, if or when such situations arise?" Appendix A, the Exercise & Sport Psychology Development Plan, provides an opportunity for personal self-reflection and goal setting.

In addition to generic issues of practitioner competence, psychotherapists including exercise and, more broadly, sport psychology, in their therapeutic armamentarium need to examine certain specific aspects of competence, including practice competence, the need for specificity of sport knowledge, and title usage.

The question of expansion into sport psychology by already-practicing therapists is one that has been addressed directly by APA's Division of Exercise and Sport Psychology in a pamphlet, *How Can a Psychologist Become a Sport Psychologist?* (APA, 1998b):

> I am a very experienced tennis player (or golfer or runner or . . .), and I am a psychologist. Can I call myself, and practice as, a "sport psychologist"?
>
> I coach (or used to coach) basketball (or soccer or football or . . .), and I am a psychologist. Can I call myself, and practice as, a "sport psychologist"?
>
> I've read quite a bit about sport psychology, and I am a psychologist. Can I call myself, and practice as, a "sport psychologist"?

The answer to these commonly asked questions is "No, none of the above would be sufficient to indicate that you are practicing within your boundaries of competence." This is an issue of both ethics and training.

PRACTICE COMPETENCE

For psychotherapists interested in supporting their clients' use of exercise, two particular areas of practice competence need to be addressed. One has to do with domains of knowledge: the prescription of exercise with clients and the use of psychological skills techniques. The other relates, broadly defined, to cultural competence.

Specific Knowledge for Therapists Using Exercise in Therapy

In addition to general psychotherapeutic skills, two domains of competence are relevant to therapists using exercise in therapy: the prescription of exercise with clients and the use of psychological skills techniques. In order to be competent in the former, it is important to have some knowledge of both the physiological and social bases of exercise and sport. Psychological skills techniques can well be acquired through knowledge of the applied sport psychology literature. Alternatively, since most of the techniques are derived from cognitive-behavioral methods in psychology, there are a number of additional avenues for accessing such information and developing skill in the use of these methods.

Cultural Competence

In a survey of members of APA's Division of Clinical Psychology, Petrie and Diehl (1995) found that whereas 96% had never received formal training or (99%) supervision in sport psychology, 20% had consulted with an athlete or sport team, and 50% had provided therapy to athletes. Although some of the contacts focused on general life issues, a significant number involved "issues in which athletic identity or sport performance were central, such as performance enhancement, depression associated with athletic injury, and disordered eating behaviors related to weight requirements or sport involvement" (Petrie & Diehl, 1995, p. 290). It is suggested here that the practitioner working with athletes needs to understand issues specific to athletes and the athlete culture (Cogan, 1998; Mooney, 1993). Within athlete culture, as well, more traditional diversity issues are relevant. For example, particularly within certain team sports, a large proportion of players are ethnic minorities, yet the vast majority of psychotherapists and sport psychologists are not and may well bring to their work their own cultural understanding of the world (Sachs, 1993). Additionally, diversity refers to gender, class, sexual orientation, and disability, among other characteristics. As I described in chapters 15 and 17, especially, these aspects of diversity are also salient to the practitioner.

SPORT-SPECIFIC KNOWLEDGE

The more forms of exercise and sport with which a therapist is familiar, the broader the range of options she or he may explore with clients interested in engaging in exercise. Although breadth of knowledge is useful, depth may be equally as important. Lack of sport-specific knowledge can be considered a competence concern in some situations. Recommendations that defy motoric capabilities or belie physiological functioning can be physically detrimental, psychologically frustrating, or both. They also can erode trust in the prescriber. If one does not already have familiarity with a particular form of exercise or sport, additional knowledge can be gained through reading, learning the rules and requirements, and observing, whether live or by video (Gould & Damarjian, 1998; Petrie, 1998; Sachs, 1993). Depending on the presenting issue, if the practitioner takes a consultative stance that imputes knowledge of the specific sport to the client and knowledge of methodologies to the consultant, the client may feel empowered, and the practitioner not overextend her or his claims of competence (Hays, 1992; Hays & Smith, 1996; Sachs, 1993).

THE HUBRIS FACTOR

The more training one has, the more impervious one may feel to the rules governing "ordinary mortals." When sport is seen as an adjective modifying the term *psychologist,* rather than a specialty designation, psychologists may assume that by virtue of their knowledge of psychology, they can practice a variant. This tendency may be exacerbated in the current marketplace of practice anxiety and diversification engendered by managed care and other contemporary pressures. A psychologist would not necessarily take lightly the modifiers "neuro-" or "forensic." Yet, the temptation may be greater when it comes to sport, since this is an area in which in one way or another many of us have participated.

When the AAASP developed a certification program, the question of title was subject to considerable deliberation. Because of the potential for violating state and provincial law if the term psychologist included those who did not meet statutory regulation, ultimately AAASP decided to designate qualified practitioners as "Certified Consultant, AAASP" (Zaichkowsky & Perna, 1996).

Confidentiality

Confidentiality is one of the cornerstones of psychotherapy, described as a "primary obligation" (APA, 1992, p. 1606) for psychologists. To a large extent, confidentiality and privacy are not compromised when the therapeutic enterprise involves exercise. A few possible exceptions are worth noting, however. As illustrated in the sidebar on page 208, one anomaly is the generally disquieting experience of encountering a client in a social setting—with the added fillip that both parties may be naked. My own experience, as the psychologist also noted, is that, with a bit of discussion, confidentiality and privacy with regard to therapy can easily be preserved.

For a variety of reasons, in real life the classical ideal of entire anonymity may be broken. Exercising while doing therapy with a client moves the dyad away from that insulated space and risks identification of the client by other people (Hays, 1994b). Informally, colleagues and I have discussed whether it would be advisable to have clients sign a waiver with regard to both liability (physical safety) and confidentiality when exercising with clients while doing therapy. This may be an appropriate option for some therapists to use. Up to now, it has not appeared necessary in my own practice. However, discussion

> Although I don't exercise with my clients per se, I often see them at the health club which I attend. Since this is a small town, I usually discuss this as a possibility that may occur so that clients can discuss and work through any feelings they may have in seeing me working out (or in the locker room). This hasn't posed a problem since the first time that I ran into a client in the locker room (and we were both fresh from showering), and I hadn't discussed the possibility as I wasn't aware that she also attended the same health club. It worked out: We both continued to work out at that club with an understanding that we barely acknowledged each other in that setting that was sacred time and place for both of us.
>
> **44-year-old female psychologist**

with each client about these potential issues may serve a prophylactic function. Such discussion may vary, also, depending in part on the size of the community and social visibility of the client.

Other, perhaps untoward, experiences that raise issues of confidentiality can also occur:

> After a complicated and abrupt termination of psychotherapy, a client called. She was upset by continuing feelings of dependency and longing that had been stirred up in particular earlier that day, when she had seen me outside walking with someone who she assumed was a client. We were able, in the telephone conversation, to process and normalize some of her thoughts and feelings.

In this example, the person feeling troubled was not the client with whom I was walking (who was, indeed, a client) but the client who was observing my actions—whether I had been seen with a client or not. Since therapists cannot predict all nontreatment situations in which they may encounter clients, the best defense may be awareness of this potentiality, as well as suitable discussion with clients if meetings occur.

Confidentiality issues have the potential to become somewhat more complex when therapists work with high-performance athletes. Some of these relate to differences in sport and therapy cultures and some to certain demand characteristics of working with high-visibility clients. Psychologists are obligated not to disclose information concerning clients except as that privilege is waived by clients (APA, 1992). In contrast, coaches are routinely quoted in the press discussing their players (Ellickson & Brown, 1990). Do psychologists' obligations to confidentiality change when they work with athletes? No, even though the temptation of disclosure to the media becomes increasingly seductive the more important or famous the client is (Sachs, 1993). The AAASP standards explicitly expect that the practitioner will refrain from disclosure unless authorized to do so in writing.

As in other systemic, contractual, or consultative contexts, there is the common ethical dilemma of disclosure if a therapist is hired by a team administrator to work with specific individuals. In a survey of AAASP student and professional members, respondents expressed particular concern about how to deal with coaches seeking information about their athletes (Petitpas, Brewer, Rivera, & Van Raalte, 1994). It is important to discuss and specify, possibly in writing, how confidentiality will be handled before such consultation begins.

Boundaries

Issues around professional boundaries, again, are endemic to any profession. Whereas the model of the therapeutic frame is useful in certain circumstances, it runs counter to some of the tradition within sport. This natural tension is important to recognize and review.

In psychotherapy practice, a number of principles underly consideration of boundaries (Smith & Fitzpatrick, 1995). These include the principles of abstinence, that is refraining from self-seeking and personal gratification; a duty to neutrality, in which the client's agenda is paramount; and the fostering of the client's autonomy and independence. One may consider this an elaboration of the guiding principle central to all ethics, that is, respect for human beings (Whelan et al., 1996).

Although the establishment and maintenance of appropriate boundaries is crucial, it is also important to recognize that (a) boundaries are regularly transgressed, (b) these transgressions are not always detrimental to the client, and (c) boundary transgressions occur along a continuum of helpfulness–harm to the client (Smith & Fitzpatrick, 1995). Boundary *crossings* (as opposed to boundary violations) is a nonpejorative term used to describe departures from accepted practice that may or may not be harmful to the client. The central question is "How can my client most benefit?" (Smith & Fitzpatrick, 1995, p. 500). In contrast, boundary *violations* are departures from accepted practice that place the client or the therapeutic process at serious risk. The complexity of even these distinctions is that on this continuum, some practices might be considered crossings or violations by practitioners of certain beliefs but not others, some crossings may compromise practitioners' objectivity or expertise, and some may contextually appear neutral to one or another party. With few exceptions, the ethical dilemmas that practitioners find themselves in are extremely complex, and subject to a variety of explanations and rationalizations.

Concerns about boundaries may take on particular significance for the already-trained practitioner newly engaging in working with clients in regard to exercise or sports (Hays, 1995; Sachs, 1993). It is especially important to note changes in the relationship between practitioner and client, and the ways in which those differences are understood and monitored. The potential for expanded engagement with the client, away from the office setting, increases the possibility for loss of traditional structures and for the adoption of a more casual relationship. Exercising with clients, observing them on the playing field (whether in practice or competition), working with high-profile clients—all involve changes from the standard dyadic in-office 50-minute hour. Therapists therefore need to monitor possible shifts in role relationships, levels of self-disclosure, and power and gender imbalances (Hays, 1994b). For any activities that may involve crossings, it behooves the practitioner (a) to think through the meaning, possibilities, constructions, and intentions of actions beforehand and (b) to have an ongoing means of reviewing these questions. Such review might occur through reflection, supervision, or consultation (Sachs, 1993).

Particular aspects of practice that involve boundary concerns include dual role relationships, self-disclosure, and physical or sexual contact. Each of these is discussed further.

DUAL ROLE RELATIONSHIPS

Dual role relationships are inherently complex. Although they may not be inappropriate, confusing, or exploitative per se, they need to be examined carefully for their ramifications. The primary question is whether there are ways in which one role relationship will interfere with, rather than enhance, the other.

In terms of role relationships as well as competence, psychotherapists using exercise in therapy need to make sure that they are acting neither as physicians nor coaches. Along with issues of competence, each profession has its own tradition, involving different and at times competing demands. Ellickson and Brown (1990), for example, suggested that there are conflicts of interest in taking on the roles, simultaneously, of coach and sport psychologist. Divergent functions include focus on the individual vs. the team, knowledge through scientific inquiry vs. social validation, assessment vs. insight, traditions of confidentiality around public statements, and the flexibility of interpersonal boundaries.

In the past few years, I have consulted with colleagues in regard to some of these complex dual role situations. Two are described below:

> In the tradition of activity therapy, a clinical sport psychologist worked with an 8-year-old boy who was not responsive to

traditional psychotherapy. The psychologist, a black belt karate instructor, taught his client a variety of kicks, breathing techniques, and relaxation, all in relation to assisting the client with impulse control. The client enjoyed the sessions and viewed the treatment as karate instruction. Was this psychotherapy? Was it karate instruction? What should he call what he was doing? What fees should the practitioner charge? Who should pay for it?

Another psychologist, employed by a boarding school, loved to play tennis. Whenever he was able, he would join the school's tennis team at their afternoon practices. He described the students as "unbelievable players. I have reverence for them." He recognized that the school culture fostered permeable and fluid interpersonal boundaries. His actions, he knew, might serve to blur some distinctions even further. Yet he justified his engagement with the team from various angles: The students were always looking for tennis partners; the coach was more comfortable with him because of this connection, and in fact at times asked him to assess student issues on an informal basis. The psychologist felt that referral relationships with these students worked out especially well because they saw him as "one of them" in this setting, rather than only knowing him through the formality of the health and counseling center.

In both these instances, the cautious therapist would avoid such challenging dilemmas. Yet it also can be argued that these are situations that allow the full range of skills for this particular therapist in this particular setting. Continual reflection, supervision, peer consultation, and discussion with the parties involved all can allow for the most effective treatment to occur.

SELF-DISCLOSURE

Among various therapeutic orientations, there are wide differences in beliefs and practices around self-disclosure (Smith & Fitzpatrick, 1995). When therapist and client exercise during therapy, the shared physical activity and sense of joint endeavor may evoke increased openness and therapist self-disclosure (Hays, 1994b; Kostrubala, 1977). In a case study of running therapy, I described an aspect of "the therapist's real existence":

> I have a minor hearing loss in one ear. In the office, I compensate well, by the angle of my head and by unconscious lip reading. These aids were less available on the road as we ran side by side, and only occasionally could I see [the client's] mouth. Traffic as well as other outdoor noises contributed to an auditory jumble. After I began to lose part of the content of a session, I recognized that I needed to disclose my handicap so that I could run with my more acute ear nearer [her]. (Hays, 1994b, p. 728)

The issue of self-disclosure also is important as it relates to the principle of (emotional) abstinence. Inappropriate therapist self-disclosure is the most frequent type of boundary violation to precede therapist-client sex (Smith & Fitzpatrick, 1995). The issue may not be that of self-disclosure, per se, but the appropriateness of the self-disclosure, in relation to the client and the situation.

PHYSICAL CONTACT (NONEROTIC)

Within and between different schools of psychotherapy and at different times in the history of psychotherapy, there has been a range of attitude toward the appropriateness of nonerotic physical contact (Smith & Fitzpatrick, 1995). Nonetheless, those are minor variations when one compares and contrasts beliefs regarding touch within therapy as compared with attitudes and behaviors within the sport world. Not wanting to appear as an awkward, aloof outsider in public settings and wanting to engage in the connections that others experience, the therapist can become swept up in the excitement and energy of competition and may well see the typical communicative expressions through touch as appropriate.

Visual contact is another form of intimacy that shifts in the setting of sport (Hays, 1994b; Sachs, 1993). People changing in the locker room, tight or revealing clothing, the effects of exertion—all form a kind of intimacy that has bounds different from the psychotherapy practice.

These may be benign in and of themselves, or benign to the practitioner, but bear meaning to the client. However, those in positions of power, whether by virtue of sex, age, status, or race, may be impervious to the meanings ascribed to their behaviors by those with lesser power (Rutter, 1986). It behooves the practitioner to attend to and understand the client's ascriptions, ensuring that the client is not harmed by even seemingly benign behaviors.

SEXUAL CONTACT

Whether the practitioner is in a position of power and authority by virtue of being consultant, teacher, advisor, administrator, or therapist, the interaction of sexual attraction, power, and dependency are of major concern (Berger, 1993; Nelson, 1994; Rutter, 1986). The most recent report of APA's Ethics Committee indicates that the largest single category of cases that resulted in loss of APA membership—67%—were cases of sexual misconduct involving adult clients. As had been noted in previous such reports, the vast majority involved male therapists and female clients (Report, 1997).

Sexual intimacy between therapist and client has been described as "arguably the most disruptive and potentially damaging boundary violation that can occur in therapy" (Smith & Fitzpatrick, 1995, p. 503). The violation of trust through sexuality by someone in authority can be markedly damaging in other power relationships as well (Berger, 1993; Rutter, 1986). Yet 23% of respondents to the AAASP survey (Petitpas et al., 1994) responded with acceptance (under many circumstances or unquestionably yes) to the item "becoming sexually involved with a client *after* [sic] discontinuing a professional relationship" (p. 143). The APA Ethics Standards specifically proscribe sexual intimacy with former clients or patients for 2 years after the termination of therapy. Even thereafter, the psychologist maintains responsibility for indicating that there has been no exploitation. In some contrast, the comparable AAASP Standards uses the APA model around exploitative relationships but implies only a current time frame: "AAASP members do not engage in sexual relationships with students, supervisees or clients over whom the AAASP member has evaluative, direct or indirect authority, because such relationships are so likely to impair judgment or be exploitative." (AAASP, 1996, p. 7).

Sexual intimacy does not occur in a vacuum. Although there are not yet specific data concerning the frequency of sexual contact by sport psychologists, there is no reason to believe that it would be less than that of other psychologists or providers of mental health services. It may be that the variations in training and professional orientation, type of client population (in performance enhancement work, typically, young, active, attractive college students), the setting, and the altered cultural norms around touching, all could predict a greater likelihood of inappropriate sexualization of the relationship (Andersen, 1994; Petitpas et al., 1994; Sachs, 1993). Thus, although the AAASP Standards may well be an attempt at judicious balancing that reflects the varying disciplines from which they are derived, I would counsel practitioners to adhere to (and value) the perspective implied in the APA Code.

Diagnosis

Concerns with regard to diagnosis, and, relatedly, psychopathology and third-party payment, may arise when licensed therapists work with people seeking services other than psychotherapy. This can be an especially murky area for the licensed clinician (i.e., someone whose psychotherapy services are reimbursable by third-party payors) engaged in psychological skills training. There are actually a number of issues embedded in such a scenario: Does the client have a diagnosable mental illness? Would the client consider clinical diagnosis stigmatizing? Would a diagnostic framework on the part of the practitioner color the practitioner's view of the client's problem and solutions to that problem? Is the client seeking psychotherapy? Are the services being provided considered psychotherapy by a third-party payor?

The clinical practitioner working in sport and exercise psychology may operate on the cusp of the wellness-illness continuum. Clients may not be seeking psychotherapy, or they may not have definable psychopathology. Although therapeutic, the services provided may not be psychotherapy. Further, it has been suggested that pathologizing normative experiences may have demoralizing effects on clients (Danish, Petitpas, & Hale, 1995). The practitioner accustomed to diagnosis and third-party billing thus confronts both ethical and legal dilemmas in considering the source of payment for services, particularly with individuals. False diagnosis for the purpose of reimbursement is unethical; however, in certain situations, especially those that are more extensive than PST, diagnostic criteria may well be met. It is prudent to think through sources of reimbursement before embarking in a particular direction. It also is important to review payment options with the contracting party (Sachs, 1993).

Ethical issues often remain dry and theoretical—until the practitioner is confronted with the challenge of enacting an appropriate response. Part of my purpose in detailing the case vignettes in this book has been to give the reader an opportunity to stand in the therapist's shoes. Sometimes this is in regard to techniques, at other times, ethics. How would you handle a specific situation? Thinking it through ahead of time can give the practitioner firmer footing when the time for action comes.

The Next Steps:
Education, Training, and Marketing

20

A lthough a trite comparison, it's an apt one: Reading a book is somewhat like embarking on a journey. As we have walked through this book together, spatially, if not temporally, the terrain that has been covered will have had varying familiarity to the reader. Those parts that were already known will have required only the lightest step. Other areas have involved more intensive exploration, perhaps including metaphoric bushwhacking among the undergrowth or side-trips on previously unexplored by-ways.

Speaking more concretely, as a result of having read this book I hope that therapists will feel knowledgeable about and inspired to support the use of exercise for their clients. Perhaps nonexercising therapists will have reflected on some of their own thoughts, feelings, and actions, and are contemplating or preparing to develop a means of regular exercise for themselves as well. With proper cautions applied, therapists may even consider whether it is beneficial to some clients to exercise during the therapy hour.

In this final chapter, I will touch on the next steps for the individual practitioner: education, training, and marketing. I will conclude with some thoughts about further areas for this field to explore, as well.

In reading the following sections, it may be helpful to review Appendix A, the Exercise and Sport Psychology Development Plan. Specific questions are raised there for individual consideration, regarding self-assessment, professional issues, office issues, financial plan, and marketing, along with an exercise and sport psychology development matrix. Here, a number of these issues are discussed in regard to two significant aspects of practice development—education and training and marketing.

Education and Training

In this section, a sometimes arbitrary distinction is made between formal graduate education and postgraduate training that may occur in a variety of ways. Education or training with regard to the prescription of exercise for psychotherapy clients is presented in contradistinction to that with regard to sport psychology, a field in its own right.

Many individuals and organizations involved in the hybrid beast that is sport psychology have a stake in the challenging issue of appropriate training to become a sport psychologist. A field that is composed of both sport science and psychology, sport psychology training and practice concerns are of interest to (a) counseling or clinical practitioners, whether psychologists or other mental health providers; (b) academicians trained in sport sciences; (c) graduate or undergraduate students trying to understand the best route to their goal; (d) university academic departments, beset by competition, downsizing, and tradition; and (e) professional organizations, establishing their turf, status, and constituency.

The primary focus of this book has been on exercise therapy, the value of exercise to the mental well-being of psychotherapy clients. Throughout, it has been suggested that the competent therapist, fully mindful of her or his ethical limitations, need not have specialized training in exercise in order to support clients' use of exercise for their own well-being. At the same time, the more information the therapist has, the more versatile she or he can be in individualizing exercise recommendations. When assisting clients to begin and maintain exercise, it is especially useful to understand motivational processes, various exercise and sport characteristics, and exercise physiology. Aware of one's own limitations of role as well as skill, the therapist can conceptualize his or her work as part of an interdisciplinary team. Potential problems can be short-circuited when the work of other professionals is experienced as complementary rather than competitive with one's own role.

Building on one's transferable knowledge and skills from other domains is vital, both in elaborating one's practice and in setting oneself apart as a provider of particular, unique services. The standard repertoire of psychological techniques used for psychological skills training includes arousal regulation, mental imagery, goal setting, and attentional control. As has been mentioned, practitioners with cognitive-behavioral training may already use a number of these techniques. Practitioners with skills in organizational development, mental health consultation techniques, and hypnosis have a solid theoretical and practice foundation that can be applied in much of this work as well. Moreover, clinical assessment, teaching skills, and knowledge of how people behave in family and other group systems becomes crucial in the consultative process.

Beyond general psychological skills, sport psychologists need to have specialized knowledge (McCullagh & Noble, 1996; Taylor, 1994). Sport sciences—exercise physiology, biomechanics, and motor learning—provide consultants with important knowledge about physiological contributions to athletic performance. Formal training is also needed in the area of nutrition and performance enhancing drugs. In working with athletes, knowledge of sport-specific terminologies, rules, assessment and intervention techniques is helpful as well (Gould & Damarjian, 1998; Van Raalte, 1998). First-hand experience of specific sport or exercise skills can be an advantage in consultation. It also is possible to gain experience and learn more through reading, observation, and discussion with athletes, coaches, and others who are knowledgeable about specific sports or skills (Gould & Damarjian, 1998; Petrie, 1998). Athletes generally are less concerned that a consultant have specific knowledge of their sport than that the consultant is open to learning the common terms used and is able and willing to help them achieve their goals. Perhaps this reflects athletes' appreciation for the practical reality that even experienced sport and exercise psychologists cannot possibly have first-hand expertise in all sports.

No matter how much knowledge sport psychologists have, they must be able to communicate their findings and recommendations in lay terms. Practitioners should speak with athletes and coaches appropriately, using proper terminology. Additionally, consultants who let go of clinical language and formality will communicate better with their clients and be rewarded with better results (Gould & Damarjian, 1998; Van Raalte, 1998).

Part of the enticement of sport psychology may be the idea that even if one couldn't hit the home run to win the World Series or execute a perfect 10 in a gymnastics event, one could at least become the sport psychologist who could teach performance enhancement skills so that these outcomes would occur. The APA brochure, *Graduate Training and Career Possibilities in Exercise and Sport Psychology* adds a strong word of caution to the romanticized vision of being able to develop a career as "psychologist to the stars":

Very few sport psychologists earn most of their income working full-time with competitive athletes. Those professionals who consult with athletes on a part-time basis usually have other employment, such as academic positions, or more traditional clinical or counseling practices in which they earn most of their income. Over the past 3–5 years, only one or two full-time positions occurred each year for people to work with collegiate, Olympic, or professional athletes, or athletes attending private sport academies. . . . Not only are these positions few in number with no dramatic increase in sight, but they generally offer less job security than other positions. At present, staking your hopes on full-time work with elite athletes appears a risky venture. (APA, 1994)

The information that follows briefly addresses both graduate and postgraduate education and training for practitioners interested in offering sport psychology services. The focus is on the individual rather than the institutional (i.e., it does not include various discussions currently occurring within sport psychology regarding the question of academic departmental accreditation).

After a brief description of graduate training in sport psychology, more extensive discussion is provided concerning training for the already-practicing psychotherapist. Whether at the graduate or postgraduate level, the practitioner embarking on further training would do well to use the certification criteria for Certified Consultant, AAASP (Zaichkowsky & Perna, 1996) as both a guide and a goal.

GRADUATE EDUCATION IN SPORT PSYCHOLOGY

The clearest statement concerning training in sport psychology is that described in the pamphlet, *Graduate Training and Career Possibilities in Exercise and Sport Psychology*. Recognizing that "a well-integrated graduate program would combine traditional psychology, sport sciences, and sport psychology," the sentence deadpans, "however few such formal programs exist" (APA, 1994). The pamphlet suggests a multidisciplinary approach to graduate education, determined in part by a person's ultimate career goals (academic, practitioner, sport science- or psychology-focused). As of the fall of 1997, 23 APA-approved predoctoral counseling or clinical psychology internship sites across the United States offered either a rotation in the athletics department working with athletes, or provided specific training experiences with athletes (Leffingwell, 1998).

Currently, the field of sport psychology is a hybrid. For the most part, students will need to do some careful mixing and matching between sport sciences and psychology to create a program suited to their needs. A Directory of Graduate Programs in Applied Sport Psychology (Sachs, Burke, & Gomer, 1998), developed by AAASP and updated on a regular basis, contains the most complete listing of such programs. It is important to note, however, that since most psychology departments do not have doctoral programs in sport psychology, the programs that are listed and courses that are available are predominantly located within sport science departments.

METHODS OF POSTDEGREE EDUCATION AND TRAINING

Ideally, the practitioner psychologist wanting to become a sport psychologist would complete a postdoctoral training year. Frustratingly, only a few postdoctoral training positions exist (e.g., at the U.S. Olympic Committee Training Site in Colorado Springs, at Ohio State University, and at Washington State University). Some individuals obtain a second doctorate; others take specific courses, in sport psychology, motor learning, biomechanics, exercise physiology, or sport sociology. Obtaining supervised experience specifically in sport psychology is another means to augment one's knowledge. Workshops and symposia provided at the annual conventions of AAASP and APA (Division 47), as well as regional and local conferences, are excellent ways of gaining information. In addition, these conventions provide informal opportunities for becoming acquainted with the leaders of this emerging field.

One also can acquire knowledge through reading. There is a vast array of journals and books in sport psychology, from popular methods of performance enhancement to detailed academic research. *The Sport Psychologist*, aimed at the applied professional, and the *Journal of Exercise and Sport Psychology*, more research focused, both provide a broad range of research of use to the practitioner. *The Journal of Applied Sport Psychology*, a member benefit of AAASP, regularly publishes special issues with specific thematic content (e.g., gender roles, sport, and exercise; team building; and sport injury). Williams' *Applied Sport Psychology* (1998) and Weinberg and Gould's *Foundations of Sport and Exercise Psychology* (1995) each contribute an accessible overview of the field, and the nearly 1,000 page *Handbook of Research on Sport Psychology* (Singer, Murphey, & Tennant, 1993) presents the most recent compendium of research in the area.

Ongoing or as-needed individual or group case consultation or supervision also is an excellent means of learning. Whether used to supplement formal training or develop or maintain competence, consultation and supervision are important ways to address ethical and technical issues as well as engage in networks of support.

Marketing

The services provided by exercise and sport psychologists vary greatly. In the broadest frame, as has been discussed throughout this book, the exercise psychology aspect of practice may involve incorporation of an exercise perspective into one's practice. The sport psychology aspect of practice generally refers to mental skills training. Any services, and any marketing, must be done within applicable ethical bounds. The reader interested in exploring issues of marketing sport psychology in more depth should review a number of recent publications on the subject (e.g., Hays & Smith, 1996; Lesyk, 1998; Wildenhaus, 1997).

Moving into a new area of practice involves selling oneself and selling one's services. Few academicians and practitioners chose their professions anticipating that they would need to become salespeople. Issues around marketing and sales may therefore feel discomfiting (Sagal, 1997). These days, however, mental health practitioners, ironically, may be at something of an advantage. For the past number of years, the erosion of clinical practices through changes in health care delivery has made it imperative for practitioners in independent practice to think along the lines of practice diversification. Thus, although they may experience distress at these changes, many of these practitioners have developed skills to adapt to current market demands.

Once the practitioner is appropriately qualified and has defined his or her uniqueness as a professional, the central issue becomes one of visibility. Personal contacts, brochures and direct mailing, use of the media, organizations and clubs, and, increasingly, use of the Internet, all are valuable methods. Described here are some considerations with regard to referral sources, increasing visibility, and financial considerations.

REFERRAL SOURCES

Developing and maintaining referral sources is a challenging and continuous process. Broadly, the primary task is to identify and cultivate potential referral sources in the local area. The practitioner expanding practice to support clients' use of exercise may focus in particular on developing connections with medical personnel (e.g., generalist physicians, sports medicine personnel, and orthopedic surgeons, wellness clinics, and dieticians). Potential sources of referral for applied sport psychology practitioners might be coaches, athletic trainers, sports medicine specialists and orthopedic surgeons, physical therapists, fitness instructors, sport and exercise scientists, and sports agents. Approaches to these colleagues varies, depending on services that may be of interest to them and those with whom they work. An introductory letter and brochure are important ingredients. However, these will have no value unless there is some level of personal contact and follow-up by phone call, office visit, or shared meal.

INCREASING ONE'S VISIBILITY

Increasing one's visibility, or going public, involves moving, literally and figuratively beyond the four walls of one's professional office toward mass media involvement and public speaking. Depending on one's comfort with the written word, print media can be an excellent way of becoming visible, whether through topical newspaper letters, guest columns, or magazine articles. Public interviews (newspaper, radio, TV) can also provide important exposure. Various organizations, such as service and civic organizations, parent-teacher organizations, and amateur sports clubs typically are hungry for speakers and will welcome relevant content. Although these occasions may or may not net direct referrals, they can be good practice for other public engagements. Such opportunities are a way in which to incorporate one's learning as well as a means of educating the public—whether about sport psychology, specific skills, or particular topical issues. The central message of this book—the psychological value of physical activity—is one that will resonate well with the general public.

FINANCIAL CONSIDERATIONS

Regular clinical services that include a component supportive of exercise may not merit any change in fee policy. Yet if one starts working with a different population segment or offering distinctive services, changes may be warranted both in source of reimbursement and in fee schedule.

Along with an assessment of the competition's services, it is important to understand the current local financial climate. One can obtain information both from comparable practitioners and from potential referral sources. If a practitioner is going to change the source of reimbursement or rate for fees, the services provided likewise should be differentiated in some significant ways.

Financial goals need to take into consideration not only potential new earnings but financial losses of various kinds as well. Along with prospective increases, one must ask oneself, what financial losses can I sustain in order to establish this aspect of my practice? Are there nontangible benefits that offset these costs?

Different segments of the sport psychology market offer varying levels of financial remuneration. To earn more, one may consider providing certain services to a specific population that can afford to pay higher fees. Professional athletes and coaches certainly are one such group. Among amateur enthusiasts, many golfers, tennis players, figure skaters, rowers, marksmen, polo players, and equestrians are more affluent; college athletes, on the other hand, may have less discretionary income to spend on mental training. People playing individual sports tend to use sport psychology services more than others (Wildenhaus, 1997), and psychological skills training is often most effective when tailored to the individual.

Workshops and team contracts may provide good remuneration. However, these may be one-shot opportunities, rather than sustained sources of income. If it is possible to use similar materials in different settings, however, the up-front costs can be diminished.

Although pro bono work does not add directly to the income stream, it does provide sport and exercise psychology services to athletes who may benefit from them and can enhance professional development and opportunities. Besides the good deed, offering free workshops and consultations to specific people or groups often leads to other paying opportunities. It may be helpful to set up an anticipated ratio of pro bono activities compared with those for which there is reimbursement. In this way, realistic financial planning can occur. In the press of everyday practice, this ratio serves as an ongoing reminder to continue marketing through pro bono projects.

Concluding Thoughts

Exercise works. It is by no means the only thing that works to support our clients' strivings toward mental health, but it is certainly a powerful, and, within the psychotherapist community at least, underused tool.

The questions of what works for particular individuals and why it works can be supported by further research. One recurrent theme has been that at the level of the individual, positive effects may be experienced even if they are not always measurable by our current methods; the dose-response relationship may be individual; and optimal matching of exercise to person may need to be individualized as well. These conclusions are not impervious to understanding through scientific method. Noting the influence of aerobic activities on psychological factors in correlational studies in which participants self-selected their activity, Seraganian suggested that experimental procedures could take this observation into account rather than experiencing it as a confound to be overcome. "On a practical level, what is being pro-posed . . . is to let the question of interest rather than scientific con-vention drive choices as to research designs" (Seraganian, 1993, p. 387). Within psychotherapy practice, it is precisely the work with individuals that allows the practitioner and client to find those matches that are efficacious.

As research and client and therapists' voices have been describing throughout this book, exercise can be perceived as salubrious by the entire range of people who are experiencing emotionally troubling times. Practitioners and researchers can explore these possibilities more systematically and continuously.

With the increased medicalization of psychotherapy, a number of medication considerations appear relevant as well. There is still much work to be done on the effective use of exercise, and appropriate cautions, for people using psychotropic medications. And although numerous studies have been conducted comparing psychotherapy and psychotropic medication, there is as yet no research comparing treat-ments in three-way design, that is, exercise, psychotherapy, and medication, alone and in combination. Complicated to conduct? Yes. Of potential significance? Yes.

The helping professions are well served by research that explores meaningful questions. And researchers, in turn, can benefit from understanding the complexity of individuals' lives and practitioners' methods. Collaboratively, we all can move forward, working it out.

Glossary: Exercise and Sport Psychology Terms

ACUTE physical activity or exercise, in contrast to **CHRONIC** physical activity, describes either **AEROBIC** or **ANAEROBIC EXERCISE** following which there may be a specific (e.g., anxiolytic or stress-reducing) effect.

AEROBIC EXERCISE, in contrast to **ANAEROBIC EXERCISE,** refers to endurance activities that are continuous and rhythmic (e.g., running, swimming, cycling).

AFFIRMATIONS are strong, positive, realistic statements about oneself that can be used in imagery preparation or during an actual event. Affirmations are often most powerful if the therapist reflects back or incorporates the client's own words or phrases.

ANAEROBIC EXERCISE, in contrast to **AEROBIC EXERCISE,** refers to exercise that is discontinuous or involves strength training (e.g., basketball, strength training, or weight lifting).

AROUSAL MANAGEMENT refers to the optimal level of physiological (tension) or psychological (emotional) arousal for a specific activity or aspect of an activity.

ASSOCIATIVE AND DISSOCIATIVE STRATEGIES are coping strategies in which one focuses on bodily sensations (*association*) or diverts one's attention from these sensations (*dissociation*).

ATTENTION TRAINING, although similar to **CONCENTRATION TRAINING,** refers to the direction of one's thoughts. Two orthogonal dimensions of attention, or attentional styles, relate to width (broad or narrow attentional focus) and direction (external or internal).

BREATHING TECHNIQUES include various methods of diaphragmatic, as opposed to thoracic, breathing. They are clustered here, as it is often instructive to offer a smorgasbord when initially teaching these techniques, so that a client can choose among those that feel most helpful.

Deep, or diaphragmatic, breathing: complete intake of oxygen and exhalation of carbon dioxide, increasing the amount of oxygen in the blood and creating a sensation of calmness. It is the cornerstone of breathing techniques.

Rhythmic breathing: in through the nose, out through the mouth.

Triangle breathing: breathe in for a count of four, hold for a count of four, out for a count of four. Triangle breathing requires greater inhalation than rhythmic breathing to sustain an eight count (hold plus exhale) and can be augmented through an image of a triangle.

Square breathing: breathe in for a count of four, hold for a count of four, out for a count of four, hold for a count of four. As with triangle breathing, square breathing requires greater inhalation; can also augment with image of a square.

Concentration breathing: focus attention on breathing itself, either through direct observation or image of a circle.

Five-to-one count: visualize the numeral 5 and inhale deeply; exhale completely; visualize the numeral 4 with next inhalation; as exhale, say to oneself "I am more relaxed now than I was at number 5," etc.

CHRONIC PHYSICAL ACTIVITY OR EXERCISE is contrasted with **ACUTE PHYSICAL ACTIVITY OR EXERCISE** to serve as a descriptor for long-term exercise effects.

COGNITIVE RESTRUCTURING refers to a number of cognitive-behavioral techniques, including:

Self-talk: the ways in which one thinks to or about oneself. In general, positive and self-supportive self-talk can be useful for skill acquisition, as an aspect of attention control, in relation to affect, and for increasing self-efficacy.

Countering or reframing: a variety of methods can be used to identify negative cognitions and replace them or offer alternative cognitions.

Thought stopping involves deliberately using a trigger (snapping a rubber band placed around one's wrist, image of a stop sign, or the word "stop") to interrupt a negative thought sequence.

CONCENTRATION TRAINING involves attention to the specific task of being engaged in the present moment.

CUE WORDS, or **MOOD WORDS**, evoke qualities relevant to the task or sport. They can be used as an aspect of relaxation or concentration. For example, the words *relax* or *calm* can be paired with diaphragmatic breathing and ultimately be conditioned. The two syllables of *pow-er* can be experienced, rhythmically, in running or swimming. The 1-2-3 waltz rhythm can be imagined as one dances into a tennis serve. Energizing mood words include *explode, charge,* or *go.*

FIT is a mnemonic acronym to describe frequency, intensity, and time (i.e., duration). FIT is both a method to increase skills and a metaphor to measure change.

Focus object describes a physical object used as a means for concentration or arousal control. Examples include imaging the word *calm* on one's baseball glove, sequencing one's preperformance golf routine while holding a blade of grass, or deep breathing to an image of a triangle while staring at one's thumb in one's lap.

Goal setting gives the client direction and context. As with cue words, goals are most effective if client-derived. Particularly helpful are goals that are related to performance rather than outcome, behaviorally specific, explicit, challenging but possible, and framed positively. It is helpful to establish both long- and short-term goals, and to develop multiple goals (addressing different competencies) or goals with multiple levels (e.g., good, better, and best).

Iceberg profile is a pattern of response on the Profile of Mood States in which a sense of vigor is elevated, whereas negative moods (tension, depression, anger, fatigue, and confusion) are reduced.

Imagery and visualization The terms *imagery* and *visualization* are sometimes used interchangeably, although imagery includes a broader sensory spectrum than only the visual element. Often, the most effective imagery takes into account as many senses as possible. Imagery can be used for *mastery* (e.g., imagining a perfect tennis match) or *coping* (e.g., behavioral rehearsal in which one deals with a less than optimal situation).

Imagery can involve the full sequence of an event or a portion of it. Creatively, the client can be directed toward changes in time (speed), intensity, color, affective intensity, and so forth. At times it is useful to image from an *internal* (that is, inside oneself looking out) or from an *external* (looking at oneself as an observer or spectator) perspective.

Inverted-U theory is a visual description of the Yerkes-Dodson principle, which suggests that performance increases as arousal increases up to a certain level, after which increased arousal results in performance decrement.

Jacobsonian or progressive relaxation is training in tensing and then relaxing muscle groups, following a specific (e.g., head-to-toe) sequence.

Kinesthetic "anchors," adapted from Neuro-Linguistic Programming, are methods designed to physically remind the person of something (e.g., relaxation) that has been learned. The SCUBA thumb-to-forefinger signal that the person is "okay" can be used to anchor a person in a sense of emotional safety.

MEDITATION has four necessary elements that include a quiet environment, a comfortable position, a mental device (e.g., a single syllable word), and a passive, receptive attitude.

MENTAL SKILLS TRAINING: see **PSYCHOLOGICAL SKILLS TRAINING**

"PEP CHEER" is designed to increase concentration. Said to oneself, it goes:
What time is it? Now.
Where am I? Here.

PERFORMANCE ENHANCEMENT TRAINING: see **PSYCHOLOGICAL SKILLS TRAINING**

PSYCHOLOGICAL SKILLS TRAINING (PST), also called *mental skills training* or *performance enhancement training,* refers to various cognitive-behavioral techniques designed to enhance performance either directly (e.g., through regulated breathing) or indirectly (e.g., through redirection of thoughts or attention).

RELAXATION TRAINING serves a number of functions: to decrease tension and manage stress on a momentary basis, to regulate one's arousal thermostat, to facilitate recovery when there is only a short time between events or when fatigued, to regulate muscular tension through differential relaxation, to distract from other thoughts, and as a precondition for other techniques, such as imagery. Methods include various **BREATHING TECHNIQUES, JACOBSONIAN OR PROGRESSIVE RELAXATION,** and **MEDITATION.**

VISUALIZATION: see **IMAGERY**

THE ZONE OF OPTIMAL FUNCTIONING (ZOF) modifies and individualizes the **INVERTED-U.** Rather than being a fixed point, optimal performance is recognized as individualized, based on the performer's preferred level of arousal at a particular point in performance.

Exercise and Sport Psychology Development Plan

A

This appendix is designed as a working document for the practitioner developing or expanding a practice in exercise and sport psychology. You are encouraged to write in it as you read through this book.

I. Self Assessment:

    A.   Strengths I have for using exercise in my practice:

    B.   Areas I need to develop; How can I develop these skills?

    C.   Goals (write out SMART goals: Specific, Measurable, Action-oriented, Realistic, and Timed):
       1. Immediate (short term):

2. Intermediate:

3. Long term (what needs to change? how will that happen?):

4. One year from today (Date:_____), how will I know that some specific aspect of my practice with regard to clients and exercise has changed?

D. Resources
   1. Human (e.g., mentors, supervisors, consultants, colleagues):

   2. Nonhuman resources (e.g., books, articles, course work):

E. What type of situation would be "over my head"? Would I refer out? To whom? If not, what type of training or support would I require?

II. Professional Issues:

    A. What methods of record keeping will I use?

    B. How will I maintain security/confidentiality?

    C. Professional development: what do I need to learn more about and how will I do that, both short term and long term?

    D. What ethical considerations do I need to be especially vigilant about?

III. Office Issues, especially if anticipating major shifts in practice:

    A. Location
        1. How accessible is my office (physical, psychological) for what type of clients?

        2. (If contemplating such practice) What logistical possibilities exist for exercising with clients during therapy?

B. Environment
   1. Are there changes in furniture or equipment that I will need?

   2. What kind of office supplies will I need?

C. What stock items do I need to have readily available (brochures, flyers, etc.)?

D. How and what will I name this business (note: ethical issues and name registration)?

IV. **Financial Plan:**

A. What new costs would be involved?

B. What balance of income and loss leader am I willing to have? For how long?

C. What do I need to learn about business management and how will I learn it?

D. Do I have a reliable system (e.g., a software program) for bookkeeping to track costs and income?

E. What fees do I want to charge for which services? Do I want to charge by the project or by the hour? Who do I anticipate will pay? When will I review this expectation?

V. Marketing, Communications, Networking Plan:

A. What are the perceived needs or interests in my community?

B. How much time (or what proportion of my time) am I willing to devote to marketing short term?

Long term?

C. An ideal client referral for me would be (including age, gender, race and ethnicity, problems, sports ability level, type of sport, referral source, individual/team/coach/parent/administrator, work setting):

D. Who do I plan to market to directly? How will I do this?

E. Who do I plan to market to indirectly? How will I do this?

F. Why would people seek me out (product, service, relationship)?

G. How do I present myself (what image do I convey) to whom?

H. What communications opportunities do I want to use (e.g., workshops, professional organizations, civic organizations, educational institutions [elementary to university])?

    I.   What is my referral network?

VI. And furthermore

    A. What other areas of performance enhancement interest me? How may I apply these questions to those areas?

    B. What am I going to do how much less of in order to implement these changes?

    C. What additional information do I need before I can begin to implement this plan?

EXERCISE AND SPORT PSYCHOLOGY DEVELOPMENT MATRIX

Write down your thoughts about ways you could address specific populations and issues. Circle those that represent skills or knowledge you already possess. Put a square around those areas in which you need more training. Place a triangle around those circles or squares that are of particularly high interest to you.

Issue

e.g., exercise, performance enhancement, motivation, injury management

Population

e.g., outpatient clients, amateur athletes, dancers

Legend:

○ = skills and knowledge I already have
□ = skills and knowledge I need to develop
Δ = high interest for me

Appendix

A Brief History of Exercise and Sport Psychology | B

Hearing the term *sport psychologist,* those unfamiliar with the field may naturally think that this is a specialization of psychologists interested in sport. To some degree this is true. Yet from its beginnings sport psychology has been a woven cloth, the warp of physical education and the woof of psychology.

The 20th-century roots of exercise psychology lie in a couple of late 19th-century studies: one that probed the effect of hypnosis on muscular endurance, and a study by Norman Triplett that included the first experimental research on the performance effects of competition (Rejeski & Thompson, 1993). "It would appear that Triplett was the first investigator to observe the adverse effects of competitive anxiety" (Rejeski & Thompson, 1993, p. 6). The interaction of exercise and mental health was first noted in a report in 1926 by Vaux, suggesting that exercise helped relieve depression (Rejeski & Thompson, 1993).

The history of sport psychology in the United States is often described as beginning in the 1920s and 1930s when Coleman Griffith, a psychologist at the University of Illinois, conducted laboratory and field research on the subject. Additionally, he consulted with the Chicago White Sox baseball team. (In fact, he was probably the first psychologist to leave academia to engage in this aspect of practice.) He also wrote books on psychology and coaching and on psychology and athletes (Singer, 1989).

Griffith was something of an anomaly, though, and there followed only sporadic interest until the 1950s, when interest developed in motor learning and other areas of academic sport psychology. Generally such research was located within physical education departments (also known as departments of kinesiology, movement sciences, human performance, or more generically, sport sciences). Clinical psychology entered the picture in the 1960s, with an initial focus on personology and the psychological management of the elite athlete.

A tremendous explosion of interest in exercise and sport psychology occurred during the 1970s and 1980s. Research, courses, and graduate programs proliferated, primarily located within sport sciences departments. Cognitive intervention techniques were applied with competitive athletes. The zeitgeist popularization of exercise, health psychology, wellness, and a holistic perspective increased the fascination with sport psychology among the general public.

The development of sport psychology organizations paralleled the growth of the field. Several organizations that addressed sport psychology from academic, research, and sport science perspectives began in the 1960s (e.g., the North American Society for the Psychology of Sport and Physical Activity [NASPSPA], the International Society of Sport Psychology [ISSP], and The Sport Psychology Academy within the American Alliance for Health, Physical Education, Recreation and Dance [AAHPERD]).

Nearly simultaneously in the mid-1980s, two organizations formed that blended the two fields of sport science and psychology. The Association for the Advancement of Applied Sport Psychology (AAASP) got its start in 1985. Diverging from the academic research emphasis of previous organizations, it addressed applied research in real-life settings. AAASP members' primary identification is evenly split between physical education and psychology, although nearly all of its presidents have come from a sport science background. AAASP is designed "to provide a forum to address applied aspects of sport psychology such as the promotion of applied research in the areas of social, health, and performance enhancement psychology" (Williams & Straub, 1998, p. 5).

In 1986, the American Psychological Association (APA) formed a Division of Exercise and Sport Psychology (Division 47). Reflecting interest in both research and practice, the division has ties to both the Science and Practice Directorates of APA. By definition, as members of APA the members of this division are psychologists, yet a number of the academic members are based within the sport science, not the psychology, departments of their universities. At the same time, recent demographic data (APA, 1998a) indicate that the majority of Division 47 members describe themselves as mental health providers and one third list themselves as employed full-time in independent practice.

It is possible to partition sport psychology in a number of ways. One is to focus on function. For many years, the United States Olympic Sports Medicine Council divided applied sport psychology into the domains of research, educational, and clinical and counseling sport psychology (Cox, Qiu, & Liu, 1993; May, 1986; Williams & Straub, 1998). Another is to distinguish between fitness (exercise) and sport (competition). Exercise psychology attends to the body-to-mind relationship, whereas sport psychology is directed toward the mind-to-body relationship. This distinction resulted in the differentiation named in the eponymous Division 47. AAASP's method of categorization has been to demarcate both research and practice into sections relating primarily to health psychology, social psychology, and performance enhancement. Yet another perspective attends to career tracks for aspiring students. In a pamphlet developed initially by APA's Division 47 and subsequently supported by AAASP and NASPSPA (APA, 1994), the graduate training and career possibilities in exercise and sport psychology are divided into four possible career tracks: teaching or research in sport sciences and work with athletes on performance enhancement; teaching or research in psychology and work with athletes; providing clinical and counseling services to various populations, including athletes; and health promotion and working with athletes but not necessarily directly in sport psychology.

Exercise History, Motivation Inventory, and Exercise Plan | C

These are open-ended questions that can be asked in whatever natural order fits the interview.

A. Current Behavior: Do you currently exercise?

YES:
1. What do you do?
2. How often?
3. How long have you been doing it?
4. When (time of day)?
5. Alone or with others?
6. How convenient or inconvenient is it for you?
7. How much does exercise matter to you?
8. How do you feel when you exercise?
9. All things considered, does this feel like the right type and amount for you at this point in your life?
10. What do you like about exercising?
11. What barriers or potential barriers are there for you?

NO:
1. Have you exercised regularly at some other time in your life?
2. Do you currently:
   a. think exercise is irrelevant and have no thoughts of exercising?
   b. think that you probably should exercise?
   c. have some interest in exercising?
   d. try to get out (e.g., take a 15 minute walk) at least occasionally?

3. Are there others in your life (family members, physician, etc.) who encourage you to exercise or would be supportive if you did?

B. Exercise History

1. Have you exercised regularly in the past?
2. What have you enjoyed?
3. What were the particularly relevant aspects (e.g., alone vs. with others, individual vs. team, self-directed vs. program, ease of activity vs. skill development, predictability vs. thrill or variability, self-focused vs. competition)?
4. Are there forms of exercise or exercise programs that you have wished to participate in or thought about learning?
5. What has been problematic? Why did you stop? How would that form of exercise/activity be difficult to engage in now?

C. Decisional Balance

The Decisional Balance Scale (next page) can assist client and therapist to understand intentions, supports, resistances, and barriers. It can be completed any number of times, with any appropriate completions of the sentence stem, "If I . . . ," e.g. "read about the benefits of exercise" or "exercise regularly."

Name _____

Date _____

Decisional Balance Scale

	Pros	Cons
1. Consequences to myself		
2. Consequences to others		
3. Reactions of myself		
4. Reactions of others		

D. Exercise Plan:

1. Relevant factors:
   a. Personal
      1) maximize self-efficacy for exercise, perceived physical competence, enjoyment
      2) maximize appropriate dimensions, including desire to be alone vs. with others, individual vs. team, self-directed vs. program, ease of activity vs. skill development, predictability vs. thrill or variability, self-focused vs. competition
      3) personal motivation (e.g., health, mental health, weight management, sociability, competence):
      4) maximize exercise type, time, etc. to relevant clinical issues
   b. Environmental (social/physical):
      maximize social support (family, peers)
      maximize access (physical access, psychological access, convenience, minimal disruption to daily life, low cost)
      time of day
2. Activity
   Mode:
   FIT (frequency, intensity, and time [duration]):
3. Goals
   (write out in SMART terms: Specific, Measurable; Action-oriented; Realistic, and Timed):
   Short term (3 goals for next 1 week to 1 month)
   Medium term (3 to 6 months)
   Long term (one year)
4. Self-monitoring
   Logging or journal writing
5. Predict relapse
   What are the most likely points of relapse?
   What are ways to counter them?

References

Acevedo, E. O. (1994). Reality therapy: A framework for implementing psychological skills for athletes. *Journal of Reality Therapy, 14,* 29–36.

Airhihenbuwa, C. O., Kumanyika, S., Agurs, T. D., & Lowe, A. (1995). Perceptions and beliefs about exercise, rest, and health among African-Americans. *American Journal of Health Promotion, 9,* 426–429.

Allison, D. B., Faith, M. S., & Franklin, R. D. (1995). Antecedent exercise in the treatment of disruptive behavior: A meta-analytic review. *Clinical Psychology: Science and Practice, 2,* 279–303.

Allison, M. T. (1991). Role conflict and the female athlete: Preoccupations with little grounding. *Journal of Applied Sport Psychology, 3,* 49–60.

Altshul, V. A. (1981). Should we advise our depressed patients to run? In M. H. Sacks & M. L. Sachs (Eds.), *Psychology of running* (pp. 50–56). Champaign, IL: Human Kinetics.

American Psychiatric Association. (1993). *Practice guideline for major depressive disorder in adults.* Washington, DC: Author.

American Psychological Association. (1992). Ethical principles of psychologists and code of conduct. *American Psychologist, 47,* 1597–1611.

American Psychological Association. (1994). *Graduate training & career possibilities in exercise & sport psychology* (Rev. ed.). Washington, DC: Author.

American Psychological Association. (1997). *Working with older adults* [Brochure]. Washington, DC: Author.

American Psychological Association. (1998a). *Employment and membership characteristics of division 47, 1997.* Unpublished report, American Psychological Association Research Office. Washington, DC: Author.

American Psychological Association. (1998b). *How can a psychologist become a sport psychologist?* (2nd printing). Washington, DC: Author.

Andersen, M. B. (1994). Ethical considerations in the supervision of applied sport psychology graduate students. *Journal of Applied Sport Psychology, 6,* 135–151.

Andersen, M. B., Butki, B. D., & Heyman, S. R. (1996). Homophobia and sport experience: A survey of college students. *Academic Athletic Journal, 12,* 27–38.

Andersen, M. B., Denson, E. L., Brewer, B. W., & Van Raalte, J. L. (1994). Disorders of personality and mood in athletes: Recognition and referral. *Journal of Applied Sport Psychology, 6,* 168–184.

Andersen, M. B., & Williams-Rice, B. T. (1996). Supervision in the education and training of sport psychology service providers. *The Sport Psychologist, 10,* 278–290.

Association for the Advancement of Applied Sport Psychology. (1996). *Ethical principles and standards of the Association for the Advancement of Applied Sport Psychology.* Unpublished manuscript.

Auchus, M. P. (1993). Therapeutic aspects of a weight lifting program with seriously psychiatrically disabled outpatients. *The Psychotherapy Bulletin, 28,* 30–31, 34–36.

Auchus, M. P., & Kaslow, N. J. (1994). Weight lifting therapy: A preliminary report. *Psychosocial Rehabilitation Journal, 18,* 99–102.

Auchus, M. P., Wood, K., & Kaslow, N. (1995). Exercise patterns of psychiatric patients admitted to a short-term inpatient unit. *Psychosocial Rehabilitation Journal, 18,* 137–140.

Bacon, V. L. (1997, September). Re-solving voice and the female college athlete. [Abstract]. *Journal of Applied Sport Psychology 9, [Suppl.],* S18.

Bahrke, M. S., & Morgan, W. P. (1978). Anxiety reduction following exercise and meditation. *Cognitive Therapy and Research, 2,* 323–333.

Bányai, É. I., Zseni, A., & Túry, F. (1993). Active-alert hypnosis in psychotherapy. In J. W. Rhue, S. J. Lynn, & J. Kirsch (Eds.), *Handbook of clinical hypnosis* (pp. 271–290). Washington, DC: American Psychological Association.

Barbach, L. (1994). *The pause: Positive approaches to menopause.* New York: Signet.

Barlow, D. H., & Cerny, J. A. (1988). *Psychological treatment of panic.* New York: Guilford.

Barnes, L. (1980). Running therapy: Organized and moving. *Physician and Sportsmedicine, 8,* 97–100.

Barrow, J. C., English, T., & Pinkerton, R. S. (1987). Physical fitness training: Benefits for professional psychologist? *Professional Psychology: Research and Practice, 18,* 66–70.

Beck, A., Rush, J., Hollon, S., & Shaw, B. (1979). *Cognitive therapy of depression.* New York: Guilford.

Benson, H. (1984). *Beyond the relaxation response.* New York: Berkley.

Berger, B. G. (1984a). Running away from anxiety and depression: A female as well as male race. In M. L. Sachs & G. W. Buffone (Eds.), *Running as therapy: An integrated approach* (pp. 138–171). Lincoln: University of Nebraska Press.

Berger, B. G. (1984b). Running strategies for women and men. In M. L. Sachs & G. W. Buffone (Eds.), *Running as therapy: An integrated approach* (pp. 23–62). Lincoln: University of Nebraska Press.

Berger, B. G. (1986). Use of jogging and swimming as stress-reduction techniques. In J. H. Humphrey (Ed.), *Human stress: Current selected research (Vol. 1,* pp. 169–190). New York: AMS Press.

Berger, B. G. (1992). Mood alteration with yoga and swimming: Aerobic exercise may not be necessary. *Perceptual and Motor Skills, 75,* 1331–1343.

Berger, B. G. (1993). Ethical issues in clinical settings: A reaction to ethics in teaching, advising, and clinical services. *Quest, 45,* 106–119.

Berger, B. G. (1994). Coping with stress: The effectiveness of exercise and other techniques. *Quest, 46,* 100–119.

Berger, B. G., Friedman, E., & Eaton, M. (1988). Comparison of jogging, the relaxation response, and group interaction for stress reduction. *Journal of Sport & Exercise Psychology, 10,* 431–447.

Berger, B. G., & MacKenzie, M. M. (1981). A case study of a woman jogger: A psychodynamic analysis. In M. H. Sacks & M. L. Sachs (Eds.), *Psychology of running* (pp. 99–111). Champaign, IL: Human Kinetics.

Berger, B. G., & McInman, A. (1993). Exercise and the quality of life. In R. N.

Singer, M. Murphey, & L. K. Tennant (Eds.), *Handbook of research on sport psychology* (pp. 729–760). New York: Macmillan.

Berger, B. G., & Owen, D. R. (1986). Mood alteration with swimming: A reexamination. *Psychology and Sociology of Sport,* 97–113.

Berger, B. G., & Owen, D. R. (1988). Stress reduction and mood enhancement in four exercise modes: Swimming, body conditioning, hatha yoga, and fencing. *Research Quarterly for Exercise and Sport, 59,* 56–67.

Berger, B. G., & Owen, D. R. (1992a). Mood alteration with yoga and swimming: Aerobic exercise may not be necessary. *Perceptual and Motor Skills, 75,* 1331–1343.

Berger, B. G., & Owen, D. R. (1992b). Preliminary analysis of a causal relationship between swimming and stress reduction: Intense exercise may negate the effects. *International Journal of Sport Psychology, 23,* 70–85.

Berne, E. (1964). *Games people play.* New York: Grove.

Beumont, P. J. V., Beumont, C. C., Touyz, S. W., & Williams, H. (1997). Nutritional counseling and supervised exercise. In D. M. Garner & P. E. Garfinkel (Eds.), *Handbook of treatment for eating disorders* (2nd ed., pp. 178–187). New York: Guilford.

Biddle, S. (1993). Children, exercise and mental health. *International Journal of Sport Psychology, 24,* 200–216.

Birrell, S. (1988). Discourses on the gender/sport relationship: From women in sport to gender relations. In K. B. Pandolf (Ed.), *Exercise and Sport Sciences Reviews, 16,* (pp. 459–562). New York: Macmillan.

Blais, M. (1995). *In these girls, hope is a muscle.* New York: Warner Books.

Bloom, M. (1998, November 2). Runners used minds, not just bodies, to reach finish. *The New York Times,* p. F4.

Blumenthal, J. A., Emery, C. F., Madden, D. J., Schniebolk, S., Walsh-Riddle, M., George, L. K., McKee, D. C., Higginbotham, M. B., Cobb, F. R., & Coleman, R. E. (1991). Long-term effects of exercise on psychological functioning in older men and women. *Journal of Gerontology: Psychological Sciences, 46,* 352–361.

Bordo, S. (1993). *Unbearable weight: Feminism, Western culture, and the body.* Berkeley: University of California Press.

Borg, G. (1985). *An introduction to Borg's RPE-Scale.* Ithaca, NY: Mouvement.

Bosscher, R. J. (1993). Running and mixed physical exercises with depressed psychiatric patients. *International Journal of Sport Psychology, 24,* 170–184.

Brackenridge, C. H. (1994). Fair play or fair game? Child sexual abuse in sport organisations. *International Review for the Sociology of Sport, 29,* 287–299.

Braden, C. J., McGlone, K., & Pennington, F. (1993). Specific psychosocial and behavioral outcomes from the systemic lupus erythematosus self-help course. *Health Education Quarterly, 20,* 29–41.

Brawley, L. R., & Rodgers, W. M. (1993). Social-psychological aspects of fitness promotion. In P. Seraganian (Ed.), *Exercise psychology: The influence of physical exercise on psychological processes* (pp. 254–298). New York: Wiley.

Bredemeier, B. J. L., Desertrain, G. S., Fisher, L. A., Getty, D., Slocum, N. E., Stephens, D. E., & Warren, J. E. (1991). Epistemological perspectives among women who participate in physical activity. *Journal of Applied Sport Psychology, 3,* 87–107.

Brewer, B. W., & Petrie, T. A. (1996). Psychopathology in sport and exercise. In J. L. Van Raalte & B. W. Brewer (Eds.), *Exploring sport and exercise psychology* (pp. 257–274). Washington, DC: American Psychological Association.

Brewerton, T. D., Stellefson, E. J., Hibbs, N., Hodges, E. L., & Cochrane, C. E. (1995).

Comparison of eating disorder patients with and without compulsive eating. *International Journal of Eating Disorders, 17,* 413–416.

Brodsky, A. M. (1986). The distressed psychologist: Sexual intimacies and exploitation. In R. R. Kilburg, P. E. Nathan, & R. W. Thoreson (Eds.), *Professionals in distress: Issues, syndromes, and solutions in psychology* (pp. 153–171). Washington, DC: American Psychological Association.

Brodsky, A. M., & Ravizza, K. (1985, August). *The clinical psychologist and the sport studies specialist: An integrative approach to working with athletes.* Paper presented at the annual convention of the American Psychological Association, Los Angeles.

Brown, C. H. (1998). Basic systems theory for the sport psychologist. [Abstract]. *Journal of Applied Sport Psychology, 10* [Suppl.], S66.

Brown, J. D., & Siegel, J. M. (1988). Exercise as a buffer of life stress: A prospective study of adolescent health. *Health Psychology, 7,* 341–353.

Brown, R. S., Ramirez, D. E., & Taub, J. M. (1978). The prescription of exercise for depression. *Physician and Sportsmedicine, 6,* 35–41.

Brownell, K. D. (1994). *The LEARN program for weight control.* Dallas, TX: American Health Publishing Company.

Brownell, K. D., & Rodin, J. (1992). Prevalence of eating disorders in athletes. In K. D. Brownell, J. Rodin, & J. H. Wilmore (Eds.), *Eating, body weight and performance in athletes: Disorders of modern society* (pp. 128–145). Philadelphia: Lea & Febiger.

Bruch, H. (1978). *The golden cage: The enigma of anorexia nervosa.* New York: Vintage.

Brustad, R. J., & Ritter-Taylor, M. (1997). Applying social psychological perspectives to the sport psychology consulting process. *The Sport Psychologist, 11,* 107–119.

Buffone, G. W. (1984a). Exercise as a therapeutic adjunct. In J. M. Silva III & R. S. Weinberg (Eds.), *Psychological foundations of sport* (pp. 445–451). Champaign, IL: Human Kinetics.

Buffone, G. W. (1984b). Future directions: The potential for exercise as therapy. In M. L. Sachs & G. W. Buffone (Eds.), *Running as therapy: An integrated approach* (pp. 215–225). Lincoln: University of Nebraska Press.

Buffone, G. W. (1984c). Running and depression. In M. L. Sachs & G. W. Buffone (Eds.), *Running as therapy: An integrated approach* (pp. 6–22). Lincoln: University of Nebraska Press.

Burks, R., & Keeley, S. (1989). Exercise and diet therapy: Psychotherapists' beliefs and practices. *Professional Psychology: Research and Practice, 20,* 62–64.

Butcher, L. A. (1993). *An exploration of the potential for use of running/exercise therapy in the treatment of post-traumatic stress disorder in Vietnam War veterans.* Unpublished master's thesis, Temple University, Philadelphia.

Byrne, A., & Byrne, D. G. (1993). The effect of exercise on depression, anxiety and other mood states: A review. *Journal of Psychosomatic Research, 37,* 565–574.

Cabaj, R. P. (1996). Sexual orientation of the therapist. In R. P. Cabaj & T. S. Stein (Eds.), *Textbook on homosexuality and mental health* (pp. 513–524). Washington, DC: American Psychiatric Press.

Carlton, E. B. (1987, August). *Parent-child play, skill development, and gender.* Paper presented at the annual convention of the American Psychological Association, New York.

Carmack, M. A., & Martens, R. (1979). Measuring commitment to running: A survey of runners' attitudes and mental states. *Journal of Sport Psychology, 1,* 25–42.

Carr, C. M., & Murphy, S. M. (1995). Alcohol and drugs in sport. In S. M. Murphy (Ed.), *Sport psychology interventions* (pp. 283–306). Champaign, IL: Human Kinetics.

Casper, R. C., & Jabine, L. N. (1996). An eight-year follow-up: Outcome from adolescent compared to adult onset anorexia nervosa. *Journal of Youth and Adolescence, 25,* 499–517.

Clayton, P. J. (1990). The comorbidity factor: Establishing the primary diagnosis in patients with mixed symptoms of anxiety and depression. *Journal of Clinical Psychiatry, 51:11 [Suppl].* 35–39.

Coakley, J. (1997). Commitment, identity, and social relationships: The social dynamics of deviance among athletes. [Abstract]. *Journal of Applied Sport Psychology 8, [Suppl.],* S1.

Cogan, K. D. (1998). Putting the "clinical" into sport psychology consulting. In K. F. Hays (Ed.), *Integrating exercise, sports, movement, and mind: Therapeutic unity* (pp. 131–143). Binghamton, NY: Haworth.

Cogan, K. D., & Petrie, T. A. (1995). Sport consultation: An evaluation of a season-long intervention with female collegiate gymnasts. *The Sport Psychologist, 9,* 282–296.

Cogan, K. D., & Petrie, T. A. (1996a). Counseling college women student-athletes. In E. Etzel, A. Ferrante, & J. Pinkney (Eds.), *Counseling college student-athletes* (2nd ed., pp. 77–105). Morgantown, WV: Fitness Information Technology.

Cogan, K. D., & Petrie, T. A. (1996b). Diversity in sport. In J. L. Van Raalte & B. W. Brewer (Eds.), *Exploring sport and exercise psychology* (pp. 355–373). Washington, DC: American Psychological Association.

Conn, V. S., Taylor, S. G., & Wiman, P. (1991). Anxiety, depression, quality of life, and self-care among survivors of myocardial infarction. *Issues in Mental Health Nursing, 12,* 321–331.

Coppel, D. B. (1998). Family context: An important source of information and interventions with athletes. [Abstract]

Journal of Applied Sport Psychology 10, [Suppl.], S66.

Coster, J. S., & Schwebel, M. (1997). Well-functioning in professional psychologists. *Professional Psychology: Research & Practice, 28,* 5–13.

Courtois, C. A. (1988). *Healing the incest wound: Adult survivors in therapy.* New York: Norton.

Cousins, S. O. (1996). Exercise cognition among elderly women. *Journal of Applied Sport Psychology, 8,* 131–145.

Cox, R. H., Qiu, Y., & Liu, Z. (1993). Overview of sport psychology. In R. N. Singer, M. Murphey, & L. K. Tennant (Eds.), *Handbook of research on sport psychology* (pp. 3–31). New York: Macmillan.

Crandall, R. C. (1986). *Running: The consequences.* Jefferson, NC: McFarland & Co.

Crowther, J. H., & Sherwood, N. E. (1997). Assessment. In D. M. Garner & P. E. Garfinkel (Eds.), *Handbook of treatment for eating disorders* (2nd ed., pp. 34–49). New York: Guilford.

Csikszentmihalyi, M. (1990). *Flow: The psychology of optimal experience.* New York: Harper & Row.

Danish, S. J., Petitpas, A., & Hale, B. D. (1995). Psychological interventions: A life development model. In S. M. Murphy (Ed.), *Sport psychology interventions* (pp. 19–38). Champaign, IL: Human Kinetics.

Danish, S. J., Nellen, V. C., & Owens, S. S. (1996). Teaching life skills through sport: community-based programs for adolescents. In J. L. Van Raalte & B. W. Brewer (Eds.), *Exploring sport and exercise psychology* (pp. 205–225). Washington, DC: American Psychological Association.

Davis, C., & Fox, J. (1993). Excessive exercise and weight preoccupation in women. *Addictive Behaviors, 18,* 201–211.

Davis, C., Kennedy, S. H., Ralevski, E., Dionne, M., Brewer, H., Neitzert, C., & Ratusny, D. (1995). Obsessive compulsiveness and physical activity in anorexia nervosa and high-level exercising. *Journal of Psychosomatic Research, 39,* 967–976.

De Souza, M. J., Arce, J. C., Nulsen, J. C., & Puhl, J. L. (1994). Exercise and bone health across the life span. In D. M. Costa & S. R. Guthrie (Eds.), *Women and sport: Interdisciplinary perspectives* (pp. 211–230). Champaign, IL: Human Kinetics.

DeAngelis, T. (1997, Nov). Menopause symptoms vary among ethnic groups. *APA Monitor,* p. 16.

Dishman, R. K. (1988). Overview. In R. K. Dishman (Ed.), *Exercise adherence* (pp. 1–9). Champaign, IL: Human Kinetics.

Dishman, R. K. (1994a). Introduction: Consensus, problems, and prospects. In R. K. Dishman (Ed.), *Advances in exercise adherence* (pp. 1–27). Champaign, IL: Human Kinetics.

Dishman, R. K. (1994b). Prescribing exercise intensity for healthy adults using perceived exertion. *Medicine and Science in Sports and Exercise, 26,* 1087–1094.

Donoghue, P. J., & Siegel, M. E. (1992). *Sick and tired of feeling sick and tired.* New York: Norton.

Duda, J. (1991). Editorial comment. *Journal of Applied Sport Psychology, 3,* 1–6.

Duncan, M. C. (1997). Sociological Dimensions. In *Physical activity & sport in the lives of girls: Physical and mental health dimensions from an interdisciplinary approach* (pp. 37–47). Rockville, MD: SAMHSA.

Duquin, M. E. (1994). She flies through the air with the greatest of ease: The contributions of feminist psychology. In D. M. Costa & S. R. Guthrie (Eds.), *Women and sport: Interdisciplinary perspectives* (pp. 285–306). Champaign, IL: Human Kinetics.

Eccles, J. S., & Harold, R. D. (1991). Gender differences in sport involvement: Applying the Eccles' expectancy-value model. *Journal of Applied Sport Psychology, 3,* 7–35.

Ellickson, K. A., & Brown, D. R. (1990). Ethical considerations in dual relationships: The sport psychologist-coach. *Journal of Applied Sport Psychology, 2,* 186–190.

Ellis, A. (1994). The sport of avoiding sports and exercise: A rational emotive behavior therapy perspective. *The Sport Psychologist, 8,* 248–261.

The emotionally disturbed athlete: A round table. (1981). *The Physician & Sportsmedicine, 7,* 67–80.

Enns, C. Z., Campbell, J., Courtois, C. A., Gottlieb, M. C., Lese, K. P., Gilbert, M. S., & Forrest, L. (1998). Working with adult clients who may have experienced childhood abuse: Recommendations for assessment and practice. *Professional Psychology: Research and Practice, 29,* 245–256.

Epling, W. F., & Pierce, W. D. (1991). *Solving the anorexia puzzle: A scientific approach.* Toronto: Hogrefe & Huber.

Epstein, L. H. (1992). Exercise and obesity in children. *Journal of Applied Sport Psychology, 4,* 120–133.

Erickson, M. H., Rossi, E. L., & Rossi, S. I. (1976). *Hypnotic realities: The induction of clinical hypnosis and forms of indirect suggestion.* New York: Irvington.

Fairburn, C. G. (1995). *Overcoming binge eating.* New York: Guilford.

Fallon, P., & Wonderlich, S. A. (1997). Sexual abuse and other forms of trauma. In D. M. Garner & P. E. Garfinkel (Eds.), *Handbook of treatment for eating disorders* (2nd ed., pp. 394–414). New York: Guilford.

Fender, L. K. (1989). Athletic burnout: Potential for research and intervention strategies. *The Sport Psychologist, 3,* 63–71.

Fillingim, R. B., & Blumenthal, J. A. (1993). Psychological effects of exercise among the elderly. In P. Seraganian (Ed.), *Exercise psychology: The influence of physical exercise on psychological processes* (pp. 237–253). New York: Wiley.

Fine, A. H., & Sachs, M. L. (1997). *The total sports experience—for kids*. South Bend, IN: Diamond Communications.

Fisher, E., & Thompson, J. K. (1994). A comparative evaluation of cognitive-behavioral therapy (CBT) versus exercise therapy (ET) for the treatment of body image disturbance: Preliminary findings. *Behavior Therapy, 18*, 171–185.

Foreyt, J. P., & Goodrick, G. K. (1992). *Living without dieting*. New York: Warner.

Foster, S. (1997). Eye movement desensitization and reprocessing for psychological recovery from athletic loss and injury. [Abstract]. *Journal of Applied Sport Psychology 9, [Suppl.]*, S59.

Freedson, P., & Bunker, L. K. (1997). Physiological dimensions. In *Physical activity & sport in the lives of girls: Physical and mental health dimensions from an interdisciplinary approach* (pp. 1–16). Rockville, MD: SAMHSA.

Freud, A. (1928). *Introduction to the technique of child analysis*. Translated by L. P. Clark. New York: Nervous and Mental Disease Publishing.

Freudenberger, H. J. (1977). Burn-out: The organizational menace. *Training and Development Journal, 31*, 26–27.

Freyd, J. J. (1996). Betrayal trauma: The logic of forgetting childhood abuse. Cambridge: Harvard University Press.

Gallwey, W. T. (1997). *The inner game of tennis* (Rev. ed.). New York: Random House.

Gallwey, W. T. (1998). *The inner game of golf* (Rev. ed.). New York: Random House.

Gauvin, L., Rejeski, W. J., & Norris, J. L. (1996). A naturalistic study of the impact of acute physical activity on feeling states and affect in women. *Health Psychology, 15*, 391–397.

Gauvin, L., & Szabo, A. (1992). Application of the experience sampling method to the study of the effects of exercise withdrawal on well-being. *Journal of Sport & Exercise Psychology, 14*, 361–374.

Gelinas, D. (1983). The persisting negative effects of incest. *Psychiatry, 46*, 312–332.

Gill, D. L. (1986). *Psychological dynamics of sport*. Champaign, IL: Human Kinetics.

Gill, D. L. (1993). Competitiveness and competitive orientation in sport. In R. N. Singer, M. Murphey, & L. K. Tennant (Eds.), *Handbook of research on sport psychology* (pp. 314–327). New York: Macmillan.

Gill, D. L. (1995). Gender issues: A social-educational perspective. In S. M. Murphy (Ed.), *Sport psychology interventions* (pp. 205–234). Champaign, IL: Human Kinetics.

Gill, K., & Overdorf, V. (1994). Incentives for exercise in younger and older women. *Journal of Sport Behavior, 17*, 87–97.

Glasser, W. (1976). *Positive addiction*. New York: Harper & Row.

Gleser, J., & Brown, P. (1988). Judo principles and practices: Applications to conflict-solving strategies in psychotherapy. *American Journal of Psychotherapy, 42*, 437–447. .

Godin, G., Desharnais, R., Valois, P., Lepage, L., Jobin, J., & Bradet, R. (1994). Differences in perceived barriers to exercise between high and low intenders: Observations among different populations. *American Journal of Health Promotion, 8*, 279–285.

Gologor, E. (1979). *Psychodynamic tennis*. New York: Morrow.

Goode, E. (1998, November 24). How much therapy is enough? It depends. *The New York Times*, F1.

Goodman, A. S., Bergandi, T. A., Morgan, D. L., & Lewis, L. W. (1996, August). *Exercise adherence in the obese*. Paper presented at the annual convention of the American Psychological Association, Toronto.

Gorely, T., & Gordon, S. (1995).An examination of the transtheoretical model and exercise behavior in older adults. *Journal of Sport & Exercise Psychology, 17*, 312–324.

Gorski, T. T. (1989). *Passages through recovery*. San Francisco: Harper/Hazelden.

Gould, D., & Damarjian, N. (1998). Insights into effective sport psychology consulting. In K. F. Hays (Ed.), *Integrating exercise, sports, movement, and mind: Therapeutic unity* (pp. 111–130). Binghamton, NY: Haworth.

Green, B. S. (1995). *Jogging the mind: How to use aerobic exercise as meditation*. Dingman's Ferry, PA: Silverlake Press.

Greenberg, D., & Oglesby, C. A. (1997). Mental health dimensions. In *Physical activity & sport in the lives of girls: Physical and mental health dimensions from an interdisciplinary approach* (pp. 49–66). Rockville, MD: SAMHSA.

Greist, J. H., Klein, M. H., Eischens, R. R., Faris, J., Gurman, A. S., & Morgan, W. P. (1979). Running as treatment for depression. *Comprehensive Psychiatry, 20*, 41–54.

Grembowski, D., Patrick, D., Diehr, P., Durham, M., Beresford, S., Kay, E., & Hecht, J. (1993). Self-efficacy and health behavior among older adults. *The Journal of Health and Social Behavior, 34*, 89–104.

Griffin, J., & Harris, M. B. (1996). Coaches' attitudes, knowledge, experiences, and recommendations regarding weight control. *The Sport Psychologist, 10*, 180–194.

Guerin, J. J. (1993). *The use of sport and exercise training for adult women psychotherapy clients with Post-Traumatic Stress Disorder*. Unpublished doctoral dissertation, Temple University, Philadelphia.

Hall, R. L. (1998). Softly strong: African American women's use of exercise in therapy. In K. F. Hays (Ed.), *Integrating exercise, sports, movement, and mind: Therapeutic unity* (pp. 81–100). Binghamton, New York: Haworth.

Harris, D. V., & Harris, B. L. (1984). *The athlete's guide to sports psychology: Mental skills for physical people*. New York: Leisure Press.

Hays, K. F. (1985). Electra in mourning: Grief work and the adult incest survivor. *The Psychotherapy Patient, 2*, 45–58.

Hays, K. F. (1987). The conspiracy of silence revisited: Group therapy with adult survivors of incest. *Journal of Group Psychotherapy, Psychodrama & Sociometry, 39*, 143–156.

Hays, K. F. (1990, December 10). Mind over marathon: Your legs can carry you only so far. *Concord Monitor*, p. B7.

Hays, K. F. (1991). Learning to trust: Rock climbing with women survivors. *Convergence*, pp. 14–15.

Hays, K. F. (1992, October). *The application of principles of mental health consultation to sport psychology consultation in medical settings*. Paper presented at the annual conference of the Association for the Advancement of Applied Sport Psychology, Colorado Springs.

Hays, K. F. (1993). The use of exercise in therapy. In L. VandeCreek, S. Knapp, & T. L. Jackson (Eds.), *Innovations in Clinical Practice: A Source Book, 12*, 155–168.

Hays, K. F. (1994a, October). *Feminist approaches to sport psychology practice: A clinical perspective*. Paper presented at the annual convention of the Association for the Advancement of Applied Sport Psychology, Lake Tahoe.

Hays, K. F. (1994b). Running therapy: Special characteristics and therapeutic issues of concern. *Psychotherapy, 31*, 725–734.

Hays, K. F. (1995). Putting sport psychology into (your) practice. *Professional Psychology: Research & Practice, 26*, 33–40.

Hays, K. F. (1996, August). *Walking the walk while talking the talk: Walking during therapy*. Paper presented at the annual convention of the American Psychological Association, Toronto.

Hays, K. F., & Smith, R. J. (1996). Incorporating sport and exercise psychology into clinical practice. In J. L. Van Raalte & B. W. Brewer (Eds.), *Exploring sport and exercise psychology* (pp.

413–429). Washington, DC: American Psychological Association.

Heil, J., & Henschen, K. (1996). Assessment in sport and exercise psychology. In J. L. Van Raalte & B. W. Brewer (Eds.), *Exploring sport and exercise psychology* (pp. 229–255). Washington, DC: American Psychological Association.

Heil, J., Wakefield, C., & Reed, C. (1998). Patient as athlete: A metaphor for injury rehabilitation. In K. F. Hays (Ed.), *Integrating exercise, sports, movement, and mind: Therapeutic unity* (pp. 21–39). Binghamton, NY: Haworth.

Heitner, K. (1998, Spring). Backtalk. *Psychology of Women, 25*, p. 12.

Hellstedt, J. C. (1995). Invisible players: A family systems model. In S. M. Murphy (Ed.), *Sport psychology interventions* (pp. 117–146). Champaign, IL: Human Kinetics.

Hendricks, G. (1995). *Conscious breathing: Breathwork for health, stress release, and personal mastery.* New York: Bantam.

Henschen, K. P. (1998). Athletic staleness and burnout: Diagnosis, prevention, and treatment. In J. M. Williams (Ed.), *Applied sport psychology: Personal growth to peak performance* (3rd ed., pp. 398–408). Mountain View, CA: Mayfield.

Herman, J. L. (1992). *Trauma and recovery.* New York: Basic Books.

Heyman, S. R. (1987, August). *Special issues in counseling and therapy with gay and lesbian athletes.* Paper presented at the annual convention of the American Psychological Association. New York.

Hoffman, P. (1997). The serotonin hypothesis. In W. P. Morgan (Ed.), *Physical activity and mental health* (pp. 163–177). Washington, DC: Taylor & Francis.

Hollander-Goldfein, B., Fosshage, J. L., & Bahr, J. M. (1989). Determinants of patients' choice of therapist. *Psychotherapy, 26*, 448–461.

Holmes, D. S. (1993). Aerobic fitness and the response to psychological stress. In P. Seraganian (Ed.), *Exercise psychology: The influence of physical exercise on psychological processes* (pp. 39–63). New York: Wiley.

Horn, T. S., & Claytor, R. P. (1993). Developmental aspects of exercise psychology. In P. Seraganian (Ed.), *Exercise psychology: The influence of physical exercise on psychological processes* (pp. 299–338). New York: Wiley.

Huang, C. A., & Lynch, J. (1992). *Thinking body, dancing mind: TaoSports for extraordinary performance in athletics, business, and life.* New York: Bantam.

Jaffee, L., & Lutter, J. M. (1995). Adolescent girls: Factors influencing low and high body image. *Melpomene: A Journal for Women's Health Research, 14*, 14–22.

Janoff-Bulman, R. (1992). *Shattered assumptions: Towards a new psychology of trauma.* New York: The Free Press.

Jones, E. (1967). *Sigmund Freud life and work: Vol. 2. Years of maturity, 1901–1919.* London: Hogarth.

Johnsgard, K. W. (1989). *The exercise prescription for depression and anxiety.* New York: Plenum.

Jordan, M. R. (1986). *Taking on the gods.* Nashville, TN: Abingdon Press.

Kabat-Zinn, J. (1990). *Full catastrophe living.* New York: Dell.

Kahn, A. P., & Fawcett, J. (1993). *The encyclopedia of mental health.* New York: Facts on File.

Kavussanu, M., & McAuley, E. (1995). Exercise and optimism: Are highly active individuals more optimistic? *Journal of Sport & Exercise Psychology, 17*, 246–258.

Kern, L., Koegel, R. L., & Dunlap, G. (1984). The influence of vigorous versus mild exercise on autistic stereotyped behaviors. *Journal of Autism & Developmental Disorders, 14*, 57.

Kirkcaldy, B. D., & Shephard, R. J. (1990). Therapeutic implications of exercise. *International Journal of Sport Psychology, 21*, 165–184.

Kirschenbaum, D. S. (1992). Elements of effective weight control programs: Implications for exercise and sport psychology. *Journal of Applied Sport Psychology, 4,* 77–93.

Kirschenbaum, D. S. (1994). *Weight loss through persistence: Making science work for you.* Oakland, CA: New Harbinger.

Klein, M. H., Greist, J. H., Gurman, A. S., Neimeyer, R. A., Lesser, D. P., Bushnell, N. J., & Smith, R. E. (1985). A comparative outcome study of group psychotherapy vs. exercise treatments for depression. *International Journal of Mental Health, 13,* 148–177.

Klesges, R. C., DeBon, M., & Meyers, A. W. (1996). Obesity in African American women: Epidemiology, determinants, and treatment issues. In J. K. Thompson (Ed.), *Body image, eating disorders, and obesity: An integrative guide for assessment and treatment* (pp. 461–477). Washington, DC: American Psychological Association.

Koeppl, P. M., Heller, J., Bleecker, E. R., Meyers, D. A., Goldberg, A. P., & Bleeker, M. L. (1992). The influence of weight reduction and exercise regimes upon the personality profiles of overweight males. *Journal of Clinical Psychology, 48,* 463–471.

Kostrubala, T. (1977). *The joy of running.* New York: Pocket.

Kostrubala, T. (1984). Running and therapy. In M. L. Sachs & G. W. Buffone (Eds.), *Running as therapy: An integrated approach* (pp. 112–124). Lincoln: University of Nebraska Press.

Kremer, D., Malkin, M. J., & Benshoff, J. J. (1995). Physical activity programs offered in substance abuse treatment facilities. *Journal of Substance Abuse Treatment, 12,* 327–333.

Kroll, J. (1988). *The challenge of the borderline patient.* New York: Norton.

Kugler, J., Seelbach, H., & Kruskemper, G. M. (1994). Effects of rehabilitation exercise programmes on anxiety and depression in coronary patients: A meta-analysis. *British Journal of Clinical Psychology, 33,* 401–410.

Kunz, J. L. (1997). Drink and be active? The associations between drinking and participation in sports. *Addiction Research, 5,* 439–450.

Lamont-Mills, A., & Pretty, G. M. H. (1997). Sport as a community of interest: An unusual relationship—sport and the community psychologist [Abstract]. *Australian Journal of Psychology, 49, [Suppl.],* 107.

LaPerriere, A., Fletcher, M. A., Antoni, M. H., Klimas, N. G., Ironson, G., & Schneiderman, N. (1991). Aerobic exercise training in an AIDS risk group. *International Journal of Sports Medicine, 12,* S53–57.

Leffingwell, T. (1998). AAASP student resources Web page: Internships. Available on the World Wide Web: http://students.washington.edu/leffingw/aaasp/internships.htm.

Lendl, J. (1997). Eye movement desensitization and reprocessing for athletic performance enhancement. [Abstract]. *Journal of Applied Sport Psychology 9, [Suppl.],* S59.

Lenskyj, H. (1990). Power and play: Gender and sexuality issues in sport and physical activity. *International Review for the Sociology of Sport, 25,* 235–243.

Lerner, M. (1994). *Choices in healing: Integrating the best of conventional and complementary approaches to cancer.* Cambridge, MA: MIT Press.

Lesyk, J. J. (1998). *Developing sport psychology within your clinical practice: A practical guide for mental health professionals.* San Francisco: Jossey-Bass.

Levine, M. D. (1998). *Gay macho: The life and death of the homosexual clone* (M. S. Kimmel, Ed.). New York: NYU Press.

Linder, D. E., Pillow, D. R., & Reno, R. R. (1989). Shrinking jocks: Derogation of athletes who consult a sport psychologist. *Journal of Sport & Exercise Psychology, 11,* 270–280.

Long, B. C. (1985). Stress-management interventions: A 15-month follow-up of aerobic conditioning and stress inoculation training. *Cognitive Therapy and Research, 9,* 471–478.

Long, B. C. (1993). A cognitive perspective on the stress-reducing effects of physical exercise. In P. Seraganian (Ed.), *Exercise psychology: The influence of physical exercise on psychological processes* (pp. 339–379). New York: Wiley.

Long, B. C., & Haney, C. J. (1988). Long-term follow-up of stressed working women: A comparison of aerobic exercise and progressive relaxation. *Journal of Sport and Exercise Psychology, 10,* 461–470.

Long, B. C., & Stavel, R. V. (1995). Effects of exercise training on anxiety: A meta-analysis. *Journal of Applied Sport Psychology, 7,* 167–189.

Lox, C. L., McAuley, E., & Tucker, R. S. (1995). Exercise as an intervention for enhancing subjective well-being in an HIV-1 population. *Journal of Sport & Exercise Psychology, 17,* 345–362.

Lynch, J. (1987). *The total runner.* Englewood Cliffs, NJ: Prentice-Hall.

Mahoney, M. J. (1997). Psychotherapists' personal problems and self-care patterns. *Professional Psychology: Research & Practice, 28,* 14–16.

Mahoney, M. J., & Suinn, R. M. (1986). History and overview of modern sport psychology. *The Clinical Psychologist, 39,* 64–68.

Marcus, B. H., Albrecht, A. E., Niaura, R. S., Taylor, E. R., Simkin, L. R., Feder, S. I., Abrams, D. B., & Thompson, P. D. (1995). Exercise enhances the maintenance of smoking cessation in women. *Addictive Behaviors, 20,* 87–92.

Marcus, B. H., Rakowski, W., & Rossi, J. S. (1992). Assessing motivational readiness and decision making for exercise. *Health Psychology, 11,* 257–261.

Marcus, B. H., Rossi, J. S., Selby, V. C., Niaura, R. S., & Abrams, D. B. (1992). The stages and processes of exercise adoption and maintenance in a worksite sample. *Health Psychology, 11,* 386–395.

Martin, S. B., & Thompson, C. L. (1995). Reality therapy and goal attainment scaling: A program for freshman student athletes. *Journal of Reality Therapy, l4,* 45–54.

Martin, S. B., Thompson, C. L., & McKnight, J. (1998). An integrative psychoeducational approach to sport psychology consulting: A case study. *International Journal of Sport Psychology, 29,* 170–186.

Martins, P., & Kaplan, H. (1997). *New York City Ballet workout: Fifty stretches and exercises anyone can do for a strong, graceful, and sculpted body.* New York: Morrow.

Martinsen, E. W. (1990). Benefits of exercise for the treatment of depression. *Sports Medicine, 9,* 380–389.

Martinsen, E. W., Hoffart, A., & Solberg, Ø. (1989). Comparing aerobic and nonaerobic exercise in the treatment of clinical depression: A randomized trial. *Comprehensive Psychiatry, 30,* 324–331.

Martinsen, E. W., & Morgan, W. P. (1997). Antidepressant effects of physical activity. In W. P. Morgan (Ed.), *Physical activity and mental health* (pp. 93–106). Washington, DC: Taylor & Francis.

Martinsen, E. W., & Stanghelle, J. K. (1997). Drug therapy and physical activity. In W. P. Morgan (Ed.), *Physical activity and mental health* (pp. 81–90). Washington, DC: Taylor & Francis.

Maslach, C. (1982). *Burnout—The cost of caring.* New York: Prentice-Hall.

Maslow, A. H. (1968). *Toward a psychology of being.* New York: Van Nostrand Reinhold.

May, J. R. (1986). Sport psychology: Should psychologists become involved? *The Clinical Psychologist, 39,* 77–81.

McCann, I. L., & Pearlman, L. A. (1990). *Psychological trauma and the adult survivor: Theory, therapy and transformation.* New York: Brunner/Mazel.

McCann, L., & Holmes, D. S. (1984). Influence of aerobic exercise on depression. *Journal of Personality and Social Psychology, 46,* 1142–1147.

McCann, S. (1995). Overtraining and burnout. In S. M. Murphy (Ed.), *Sport psychology interventions* (pp. 347–368). Champaign, IL: Human Kinetics.

McCullagh, P., & Noble, J. M. (1996). Education and training in sport and exercise psychology. In J. L. Van Raalte & B. W. Brewer (Eds.), *Exploring sport and exercise psychology* (pp. 377–394). Washington, DC: American Psychological Association.

McDonald, D. G., & Hodgdon, J. A. (1991). *The psychological effects of aerobic fitness training: Research & theory.* New York: Springer-Verlag.

McEntee, D. J., & Halgin, R. P. (1996). Therapists' attitudes about addressing the role of exercise in psychotherapy. *Journal of Clinical Psychology, 52,* 48–60.

McGowan, R. W., & Pierce, E. F. (1991). Mood alterations with a single bout of physical activity. *Perceptual and Motor Skills, 72,* 1203–1209.

McGrath, E., Keita, G. P., Strickland, B. R., & Russo, N. F. (1990). *Women and depression.* Washington, DC: American Psychological Association.

McNair, D. M., Lorr, M., & Droppleman, L. F. (1971). *Profile of mood states manual.* San Diego: Educational and Industrial Testing Service.

Mehlenbeck, R. S., Coleman, J. K., Meyers, A. W., & Whelan, J. P. (1997, August). *Earning a living in sport psychology: Is anyone doing it?* Poster session presented at the annual convention of the American Psychological Association, Chicago.

Meichenbaum, D. H., & Turk, D. C. (1987). *Facilitating treatment adherence.* New York: Plenum.

Menapace, N., & Stern, E. M. (1998). Contact improvisation: Its potentials for a therapy of movement. In K. F. Hays (Ed.), *Integrating Exercise, Sports, Movement, and Mind* (pp. 41–46). Binghamton, NY: Haworth.

Meyers, A. W. (1995). Ethical principles of the Association for the Advancement of Applied Sport Psychology. *AAASP Newsletter, 10,* 15, 21.

Meyers, A. W., Whelan, J. P., & Murphy, S. (1995). Cognitive behavioral strategies in athletic performance enhancement. In M. Hersen, R. M. Eisler, & P. M. Miller (Eds.), *Progress in behavior modification* (pp. 137–164). Pacific Grove, CA: Brooks/Cole.

Miller, W. R., & Brown, S. A. (1997). Why psychologists should treat alcohol and drug problems. *American Psychologist, 52,* 1269–1279.

Mitchell, J. E., Specker, S., & Edmonson, K. (1997). Management of substance abuse and dependence. Diagnostic issues. In D. M. Garner & P. E. Garfinkel (Eds.), *Handbook of treatment for eating disorders* (2nd ed., pp. 415–423). New York: Guilford.

Mondin, G. W., Morgan, W. P., Piering, P. N., Stegner, A. J., Stotesbery, C. L., Trine, M. R., & Wu, M. Y. (1996). Psychological consequences of exercise deprivation in habitual exercisers. *Medicine & Science in Sports and Exercise, 28,* 1199–1203.

Mooney, D. K. (1993, August). *Counseling athletes: The need for a multicultural perspective.* Paper presented at the annual convention of the American Psychological Association, Toronto.

Morgan, L. K., Griffin, J., & Heyward, V. H. (1996). Ethnicity, gender, and experience effects on attributional dimensions. *The Sport Psychologist, 10,* 4–16.

Morgan, W. P. (1985a). Affective beneficence of vigorous physical activity. *Medicine and Science in Sports and Exercise, 17,* 94–100.

Morgan, W. P. (1985b). Selected psychological factors limiting performance: A mental health model. In D. H. Clarke & H. M. Eckert (Eds.), *Limits of human performance* (pp. 70–80). Champaign, IL: Human Kinetics.

Morgan, W. P. (1993). Hypnosis and sport psychology. In J. W. Rhue, S. J. Lynn, & I. Kirsch (Eds.), *Handbook of clinical hypnosis* (pp. 649–670). Washington, DC: American Psychological Association.

Morgan, W. P. (Ed.). (1997). *Physical activity and mental health*. Washington, DC: Taylor & Francis.

Morgan, W. P., Costill, D. L., Flynn, M. G., Raglin, J. S., & O'Connor, P. J. (1988). Mood disturbance following increased training in swimmers. *Medicine & Science in Sports & Exercise, 20,* 408–414.

Morgan, W. P., & Goldston, S. E. (Eds.). (1987). *Exercise and mental health*. New York: Hemisphere.

Morgan, W. P., O'Connor, P. J., Sparling, P. B., & Pate, R. R. (1987). Psychological characterization of the elite female distance runner. *International Journal of Sports Medicine, 8,* 124–131.

Morris, M., Steinberg, H., Sykes, E. A., & Salmon, P. (1990). Effects of temporary withdrawal from regular running. *Journal of Psychosomatic Research, 34,* 493–500.

Murphy, M., & White, R. A. (1995). *In the zone* (Rev. ed.). New York: Penguin.

Murphy, S. M. (1995). Transitions in competitive sport: Maximizing individual potential. In S. M. Murphy (Ed.), *Sport psychology interventions* (pp. 331–346). Champaign, IL: Human Kinetics.

Murphy, S. M. (1996). *The achievement zone*. New York: Putnam's.

Murphy, T. J., Pagano, R. R., & Marlatt, G. A. (1986). Lifestyle modification with heavy alcohol drinkers: Effects of aerobic exercise and meditation. *Addictive Behaviors, 11,* 175–186.

National Advisory Mental Health Council. (1990). *National plan for research on child and adolescent mental disorders*. (DHHS Publication No. ADM 90–1683). Washington, DC: U.S. Government Printing Office.

Nelson, M. B. (1994). *The stronger women get, the more men love football*. New York: Avon.

Norcross, J. C., Alford, B. A., & DeMichele, J. T. (1992). The future of psychother-apy: Delphi data and concluding observations. *Psychotherapy, 29,* 150–158.

North, T. C. (1997). Eye movement desensitization and reprocessing and mental training to overcome the choking response in athletics. [Abstract]. *Journal of Applied Sport Psychology 9, [Suppl.],* S58.

North, T. C., McCullagh, P., & Tran, Z. V. (1990). Effect of exercise on depression. *Exercise and Sport Sciences Reviews, 18,* 379–415.

O'Connor, P. J., & Davis, J. C. (1992). Psychobiologic responses to exercise at different times of day. *Medicine and Science in Sports and Exercise, 24,* 714–719.

Oglesby, C. A. (1995). Alternative strategies for dealing with trauma and TRAUMA in sport. [Abstract]. *Journal of Applied Sport Psychology 7, [Suppl.],* S23.

Oglesby, C. A., & Hill, K. L. (1990, August). *A family systems approach to team building in sport*. Paper presented at the annual convention of the American Psychological Association, Boston.

Oglesby, C. A., & Hill, K. L. (1993). Gender and sport. In R. B. Singer, M. Murphey, & L. K. Tennant (Eds.), *Handbook of research on sport psychology* (pp. 718–728). New York: Macmillan.

O'Hanlon, W. H., & Weiner-Davis, M. (1989). *In search of solutions: A new direction in psychotherapy*. New York: Norton.

Orwin, A. (1973). "The running treatment": A preliminary communication on a new use for an old therapy (physical activity) in the agoraphobic syndrome. *British Journal of Psychiatry, 122,* 175–179.

Ossip-Klein, D. J., Doyne, E. J., Bowman, E. D., Osborn, K. M., McDougall-Wilson, I. B., & Neimeyer, R. A. (1989). Effects of running or weight lifting on self-concept in clinically depressed women. *Journal of Consulting & Clinical Psychology, 57,* 158–161.

Pelham, T. W., & Campagna, P. D. (1991). Benefits of exercise in psychiatric rehabilitation of persons with schizophrenia.

Canadian Journal of Rehabilitation, 4, 159–168.

Pelham, T. W., Campagna, P. D., Ritvo, P. G., & Birnie, W. A. (1993). The effects of exercise therapy on clients in a psychiatric rehabilitation program. *Psychosocial Rehabilitation Journal, 16*, 75–84.

Pender, N. J., Sallis, J. F., Long, B. J., & Calfas, K. J. (1994). Health-care provider counseling to promote physical activity. In R. K. Dishman (Ed.), *Advances in exercise adherence* (pp. 213–235). Champaign, IL: Human Kinetics.

Perlman, S. G., Connell, K. J., Clark, A., Robinson, M. S., Conlon, P., Gecht, M., Caldron, P., & Sinacore, J. M. (1990). Dance-based aerobic exercise for rheumatoid arthritis. *Arthritis Care and Research, 3*, 29–35.

Petitpas, A., Brewer, B., Rivera, P., & Van Raalte, J. (1994). Ethical beliefs and behaviors in applied sport psychology: The AAASP ethics survey. *Journal of Applied Sport Psychology, 6*, 135–151.

Petrie, T. A. (1998). Anxiety management and the elite athlete: A case study. In K. F. Hays (Ed.), *Integrating exercise, sports, movement, and mind: Therapeutic unity* (pp. 161–173). Binghamton, NY: Haworth.

Petrie, T. A. (1996). Differences between male and female college lean sport athletes, nonlean sport athletes, and nonathletes on behavioral and psychological indices of eating disorders. *Journal of Applied Sport Psychology, 8*, 218–230.

Petrie, T. A., & Diehl, N. S. (1995). Sport psychology in the profession of psychology. *Professional Psychology: Research & Practice, 26*, 288–291.

Petrie, T. A., & Stoever, S. (1993). The incidence of bulimia nervosa and pathogenic weight control behaviors in female collegiate gymnasts. *Research Quarterly for Exercise and Sport, 64*, 238–241.

Petruzello, S. J., & Landers, D. M. (1994). Varying the duration of acute exercise: Implications for changes in affect. *Anxiety, Stress and Coping: An International Journal, 6*, 301–310.

Physical activity & sport in the lives of girls: Physical and mental health dimensions from an interdisciplinary approach. (1997) Rockville, MD: SAMHSA.

Pierce, R. A. (1969). Athletes in psychotherapy: How many, how come? *Journal of the American College Health Association, 17*, 244–249.

Pincus, H. A., Tanielian, T. L., Marcus, S. C., Olfson, M., Zarin, D. A., Thompson, J., & Zito, J. M. (1998). Prescribing trends in psychotropic medications: Primary care, psychiatry, and other medical specialties. *Journal of the American Medical Association, 279*, 526–531.

Pinto, B. M. (1994, May). *Women's exercise behavior. Psychosocial and behavioral factors in women's health: Creating an agenda for the 21st century.* Washington, DC: American Psychological Association.

Pinto, B. M., & Marcus, B. H. (1994). Physical activity, exercise, and cancer in women. *Medicine, Exercise, Nutrition, and Health, 3*, 102–111.

Pope, K. S., & Brown, L. S. (1996). *Recovered memories of abuse: Assessment, therapy, forensics.* Washington, DC: American Psychological Association.

Powell, R. R. (1974). Psychological effects of exercise therapy upon institutionalized geriatric mental patients. *Journal of Gerontology, 29*, 157–161.

Powers, J. M., Woody, G. E., & Sachs, M. L. (1999). Perceived effects of exercise and sport in a population defined by their injection drug use. *American Journal on Addictions, 8*, 71–75.

Prior, J. C., Gill, K., & Vigna, Y. M. (1995). Fluoxetine for premenstrual dysphoria. *The New England Journal of Medicine, 333*, 1152.

Prochaska, J. O. (1996, November). *A revolution in health promotion: How unhealthy lifestyles can be changed.* Paper presented at Frontiers of Knowledge, Concord, New Hampshire.

Prochaska, J. O., & Marcus, B. H. (1994). The transtheoretical model: Applications to exercise. In R. K. Dishman (Ed.), *Advances in exercise adherence* (pp. 161–180). Champaign, IL: Human Kinetics.

Prochaska, J. O., Norcross, J. C., & DiClemente, C. C. (1994). *Changing for good.* New York: William Morrow.

Raglin, J. S. (1990). Exercise and mental health: Beneficial and detrimental effects. *Sports Medicine, 9,* 323–329.

Raglin, J. S. (1993). Overtraining and staleness: Psychometric monitoring of endurance athletes. In R. B. Singer, M. Murphey, & L. K. Tennant (Eds.), *Handbook of research on sport psychology* (pp. 840–850). New York: Macmillan.

Raglin, J. S. (1997). Anxiolytic effects of physical activity. In W. P. Morgan (Ed.), *Physical activity and mental health* (pp. 107–126). Washington, DC: Taylor & Francis.

Rejeski, W. J., & Thompson, A. (1993). Historical and conceptual roots of exercise psychology. In P. Seraganian (Ed.), *Exercise psychology: The influence of physical exercise on psychological processes* (pp. 3–35). New York: Wiley.

Rejeski, W. J., Thompson, A., Brubaker, P. H., & Miller, H. S. (1992). Acute exercise: Buffering psychosocial stress responses in women. *Health Psychology, 11,* 355–362.

Report of the Ethics Committee, 1996. (1997). *American Psychologist, 52,* 897–905.

Reynolds, F. (1996). Working with movement as a metaphor: Understanding the therapeutic impact of physical exercise from a Gestalt perspective. *Counselling Psychology Quarterly, 9,* 383–390.

Rich, F. (1997, May 1). Journal: Harnisch's perfect pitch. *New York Times,* p. A27.

Rindskopf, K. D., & Gratch, S. E. (1982). Women and exercise: A therapeutic approach. *Women & Therapy, 1,* 15–26.

Robison, J. I., & Rogers, M. A. (1995). Impact of behavior management programs on exercise adherence. *American Journal of Health Promotion, 9,* 379–382.

Rodin, J. (1992). *Body traps: Breaking the binds that keep you from feeling good about your body.* New York: Quill.

Rodin, J., Silberstein, L. R., & Striegel-Moore, R. H. (1984). Women and weight: A normative discontent. In T. B. Sonderegger (Ed.), *Nebraska Symposium on Motivation: Vol. 32. Psychology and Gender* (pp. 267–307). Lincoln: University of Nebraska Press.

Rose, B., Larkin, D., & Berger, B. G. (1994). Perceptions of social support in children of low, moderate, and high levels of coordination. *The ACHPER Healthy Lifestyles Journal, Summer,* 18–21.

Rotella, R. J., & Murray, M. (1991). Homophobia, the world of sport, and sport psychology consulting. *The Sport Psychologist, 5,* 355–364.

Royak-Schaler, R., & Feldman, R. H. (1984). Health behaviors of psychotherapists. *Journal of Clinical Psychology, 40,* 705–710.

Rudolph, D. L., & McAuley, E. (1996). Self-efficacy and perceptions of effort: A reciprocal relationship. *Journal of Sport & Exercise Psychology, 18,* 216–223.

Runner's World presents the 1987 New York City Marathon preview. (1987). *Runner's World, 22,* 58.

Rutter, P. (1986). *Sex in the forbidden zone: When men in power—therapists, doctors, clergy, teachers, and others—betray women's trust.* Los Angeles: Tarcher.

Ryan, J. (1995). *Little girls in pretty boxes: The making and breaking of elite gymnasts and figure skaters.* New York: Doubleday.

Sachs, M. L. (1981). Running addiction. In M. H. Sacks & M. L. Sachs (Eds.), *Psychology of running* (pp. 116–126). Champaign, IL: Human Kinetics.

Sachs, M. L. (1982). Change agents in the psychology of running. In R. C. Cantu & W. J. Gillespie (Eds.), *Sports medicine, sports science: Bridging the gap* (pp. 17–26). Lexington, MA: Collamore Press.

Sachs, M. L. (1984a). The mind of the runner: Cognitive strategies used during running. In M. L. Sachs & G. W. Buffone (Eds.), *Running as therapy: An integrated approach* (pp. 288–303). Lincoln: University of Nebraska Press.

Sachs, M. L. (1984b). Psychological well-being and vigorous physical activity. In J. M. Silva III & R. S. Weinberg (Eds.), *Psychological foundations of sport* (pp. 435–444). Champaign, IL: Human Kinetics.

Sachs, M. L. (1984c). The runner's high. In M. L. Sachs & G. W. Buffone (Eds.), *Running as therapy: An integrated approach* (pp. 273–287). Lincoln: University of Nebraska Press.

Sachs, M. L. (1993). Professional ethics in sport psychology. In R. N. Singer, M. Murphey, & L. K. Tennant (Eds.), *Handbook of research on sport psychology* (pp. 921–932). New York: Macmillan.

Sachs, M. L., & Buffone, G. W. (Eds.). (1984). *Running as therapy: An integrated approach*. Lincoln: University of Nebraska Press.

Sachs, M. L., Burke, K. L., & Gomer, S. (1998). *Directory of graduate programs in applied sport psychology* (5th ed.). Morgantown, WV: FIT.

Sachs, M. L., & Pargman, D. (1984). Running addiction. In M. L. Sachs & G. W. Buffone (Eds.), *Running as therapy: An integrated approach* (pp. 231–252). Lincoln: University of Nebraska Press.

Sacks, M. H. (1981). Running addiction: A clinical report. In M. H. Sacks & M. L. Sachs (Eds.), *Psychology of running* (pp. 127–130). Champaign, IL: Human Kinetics.

Sacks, M. H., & Sachs, M. L. (Eds.). (1981). *Psychology of running*. Champaign, IL: Human Kinetics.

Sagal, M. (1997, September). The business of sport psychology consulting. *Journal of Applied Sport Psychology [Suppl.], 9,* S109.

Sallis, J. F., Simons-Morton, B. G., Stone, E. J., Corbin, C. B., Epstein, L. H., Faucette, N., Iannotti, R. J., Killen, J. D., Klesges, R. C., Petray, C. K., Rowland, T. W., & Taylor, W. C. (1992). Determinants of physical activity and interventions in youth. *Medicine and Science in Sports and Exercise, [Suppl.] 24,* S192–S195.

Schmelzer, G. L. (1996, October). Narrative means to performance enhancement ends: The use of narrative therapy in applied sport psychology. *Journal of Applied Sport Psychology [Suppl.], 8,* S125.

Seheult, C. (1997). Freud on fencing: The role of unconscious psychological defences. In R. J. Butler (Ed.), *Sports psychology in performance* (pp. 217–247). Oxford, England: Buttenworth Heinemann.

Seligman, M. E. P. (1991). *Learned optimism.* New York: Knopf.

Selye, H. (1975). *Stress without distress.* New York: Signet.

Seraganian, P. (1993). Current status and future directions in the field of exercise psychology. In P. Seraganian (Ed.), *Exercise psychology: The influence of physical exercise on psychological processes* (pp. 383–390). New York: Wiley.

Serlin, I., & Stern, E. M. (1998). The dialogue of movement. In K. F. Hays (Ed.), *Integrating Exercise, Sports, Movement, and Mind* (pp. 47–52). Binghamton, NY: Haworth.

Sheehan, G. (1978). *Running and being: The total experience.* New York: Warner Books.

Sheehan, G. (1996). *Going the distance: One man's journey to the end of his life.* New York: Villard.

Shephard, R. J. (1990). The scientific basis of exercise prescribing for the very old. *Journal of the American Geriatrics Society, 38,* 62–70.

Shipman, W. M. (1984). Emotional and behavioral effects of long-distance running on children. In M. L. Sachs & G. W. Buffone (Eds.), *Running as therapy: An integrated approach* (pp. 125–137). Lincoln: University of Nebraska Press.

Silva, J. M. (1990). An analysis of the training stress syndrome in competitive athletics. *Journal of Applied Sport Psychology, 2,* 5–20.

Silva, J. M. (1994). Sport performance phobias. *International Journal of Sport Psychology, 25,* 100–118.

Sime, W. E. (1984). Psychological benefits of exercise training in the healthy individual. In J. D. Matarazzo, S. M. Weiss, J. A. Herd, N. E. Miller, & S. M. Weiss (Eds.). *Behavioral health* (pp. 488–508). New York: Wiley.

Sime, W. E. (1996). Guidelines for clinical applications of exercise therapy for mental health. In J. L. Van Raalte & B. W. Brewer (Eds.), *Exploring sport and exercise psychology* (pp. 159–187). Washington, DC: American Psychological Association.

Sime, W. E., & Sanstead, M. (1987). Running therapy in the treatment of depression: Implications for prevention. In R. F. Munoz (Ed.), *Depression prevention* (pp. 125–138). New York: Hemisphere.

Simons, C. W., & Birkimer, J. C. (1988). An exploration of factors predicting the effects of aerobic conditioning on mood state. *Journal of Psychosomatic Research, 32,* 63–75.

Singer, R. N. (1989). Applied sport psychology in the United States. *Journal of Applied Sport Psychology, 1,* 61–80.

Singer, R. N., Murphey, M., & Tennant, L. K. (Eds.). (1993). *Handbook of research on sport psychology.* New York: Macmillan.

Sinyor, D., Brown, T., Rostant, L., & Seraganian, P. (1982). The role of a physical fitness program in the treatment of alcoholism. *Journal of Studies on Alcohol, 43,* 380–386.

Skrinar, G. S., Unger, K. V., Hutchinson, D. S., & Faigenbaum, A. D. (1992). Effects of exercise training in young adults with psychiatric disabilities. *Canadian Journal of Rehabilitation, 5,* 151–157.

Smith, R. C., & Darling, N. (1997, August). *Extracurricular activity participation as a buffer against stress and adversity.* Poster session presented at the annual meeting of the American Psychological Association, Chicago.

Smith, D., & Fitzpatrick, M. (1995). Patient-therapist boundary issues: An integrative review of theory and research. *Professional Psychology: Research and Practice, 26,* 499–506.

Smith, R. E. (1986). Toward a cognitive-affective model of athletic burnout. *Journal of Sport Psychology, 8,* 36–50.

Smith, R. E., & Smoll, F. L. (1996). Psychosocial interventions in youth sport. In J. L. Van Raalte & B. W. Brewer (Eds.), *Exploring sport and exercise psychology* (pp. 287–315). Washington, DC: American Psychological Association.

Sonstroem, R. J. (1997). Physical activity and self-esteem. In W. P. Morgan (Ed.), *Physical activity and mental health* (pp. 127–143). Washington, DC: Taylor & Francis.

Stainback, R. D., & LaMarche, J. A. (1998). Family systems issues affecting athletic performance in youth. In K. F. Hays (Ed.), *Integrating Exercise, Sports, Movement, and Mind* (pp. 5–20). Binghamton, NY: Haworth.

Steege, J. F., & Blumenthal, J. A. (1993). The effects of aerobic exercise on premenstrual symptoms in middle-aged women: A preliminary study. *Journal of Psychosomatic Research, 37,* 127–133.

Stephenson, M. G., Levy, A. S., Sass, M. L., & McGarvey, W. E. (1987). 1985 NHIS findings: Nutrition knowledge and baseline data for the weight-loss objectives. *Public Health Report, 102,* 61–67.

Steptoe, A., & Cox, S. (1988). Acute effects of aerobic exercise on mood. *Health Psychology, 7,* 329–340.

Steptoe, A., Moses, J., Edwards, S., & Mathews, A. (1993). Exercise and responsivity to mental stress: Discrepancies between the subjective and physiological effects of aerobic training. *International Journal of Sport Psychology, 24,* 110–129.

Stevenson, J. S., & Topp, R. (1990). Effects of moderate and low intensity long-term exercise by older adults. *Research in Nursing and Health, 13,* 209–218.

Strean, W. B. (1995). Youth sport contexts: Coaches' perceptions and implications for intervention. *Journal of Applied Sport Psychology, 7,* 23–37.

Strean, W. B., & Strean, H. S. (1998). Applying psychodynamic concepts to sport psychology practice. *The Sport Psychologist, 12,* 208–222.

Stein, J. M., Papp, L. A., Klein, D. F., Cohen, S., Simon, J., Ross, D., Martinez, J., & Gorman, J. M. (1992). Exercise tolerance in panic disorder patients. *Biological Psychiatry, 32,* 281–287.

Striegel-Moore, R. H., Silberstein, L. R., & Rodin, J. (1986). Toward an understanding of risk factors for bulimia. *American Psychologist, 41,* 246–263.

Suinn, R. M. (1986). *Seven steps to peak performance.* Toronto: Hans Huber.

Summers, J., & Wolstat, H. (1984). Creative running. In M. L. Sachs, & G. W. Buffone (Eds.), *Running as therapy: An integrated approach* (pp. 93–100). Lincoln: University of Nebraska Press.

A supporting cast of thousands. (1997, June 19). *Concord Monitor,* p. C7.

Swoap, R. A., & Murphy, S. M. (1995). Eating disorders and weight management in athletes. In S. M. Murphy (Ed.), *Sport psychology interventions* (pp. 307– 329). Champaign, IL: Human Kinetics.

Taylor, J. (1994). Examining the boundaries of sport science and psychology trained practitioners in applied sport psychology: Title usage and area of competence. *Journal of Applied Sport Psychology, 6,* 185–195.

Taylor, J. (1996). Intensity regulation and athletic performance. In J. L. Van Raalte & B. W. Brewer (Eds.), *Exploring sport and exercise psychology* (pp. 75–106).

Washington, DC: American Psychological Association.

Thayer, R. E., Newman, J. R., & McClain, T. M. (1994). Self-regulation of mood: strategies for changing a bad mood, raising energy, and reducing tension. *Journal of Personality and Social Psychology, 67,* 910–925.

Thompson, J. K. (1996). Introduction: Body image, eating disorders, and obesity—An emerging synthesis. In J. K. Thompson (Ed.), *Body image, eating disorders, and obesity: An integrative guide for assessment and treatment* (pp. 1–20). Washington, DC: American Psychological Association.

Thompson, R. A. (1993, August). *Excessive exercise in the athlete: A hidden eating disorder symptom.* Paper presented at the annual convention of the American Psychological Association, Toronto.

Thompson, R. A., & Sherman, R. T. (1993). *Helping athletes with eating disorders.* Champaign, IL: Human Kinetics.

Too few people are treated for depression. (1997, March). *APA Monitor, 29,* p. 6.

Turner, J. (1998, June 20). Celebrating life. *The Toronto Star,* pp. L1–L2.

Udry, E. M. (1992). Interventions for the anxious and depressed: Suggested links between control theory and exercise therapy. *Journal of Reality Therapy, 12,* 32–36.

Unger, K. V., Skrinar, G. S., Hutchinson, D. S., & Yelmokas, A. M. (1992). Fitness: A viable adjunct to treatment for young adults with psychiatric disabilities. *Psychosocial Rehabilitation Journal, 15,* 21–28.

United States Department of Health and Human Services. (1996). *Physical Activity and Health: A Report of the Surgeon General.* Atlanta, GA: U.S. Department of Health and Human Services, Centers for Disease Control and Prevention, National Center for Chronic Disease Prevention and Health Promotion.

Van Dixhoorn, J., Duivenvoorden, H. J., Pool, J., & Verhage, F. (1990). Psychic effects of physical training and relaxation therapy after myocardial infarction. *Journal of Psychosomatic Research, 34,* 327–337.

Van Raalte, J. L. (1998). Working in competitive sport: What coaches and athletes want psychologists to know. In K. F. Hays (Ed.), *Integrating exercise, sports, movement, and mind* (pp. 101–110). Binghamton, NY: Haworth.

Van Raalte, J. L., & Brewer, B. W. (Eds.). (1996). *Exploring sport and exercise psychology.* Washington, DC: American Psychological Association.

Waddell, T., & Schaap, D. (1996). *Gay Olympian: The life and death of Dr. Tom Waddell.* New York: Knopf.

Walsh, B. T., & Garner, D. M. (1997). Diagnostic issues. In D. M. Garner & P. E. Garfinkel (Eds.), *Handbook of treatment for eating disorders* (2nd ed., pp. 25–33). New York: Guilford.

Wankel, L. M. (1993). The importance of enjoyment to adherence and psychological benefits from physical activity. *International Journal of Sport Psychology, 24,* 151–169.

Weinberg, R. S., & Gould, D. (1995). *Foundations of sport and exercise psychology.* Champaign, IL: Human Kinetics.

Weiss, M. R. (1995). Children in sport: An educational model. In S. M. Murphy (Ed.), *Sport psychology interventions* (pp. 39–69). Champaign, IL: Human Kinetics.

Weiss, R. S. (1975). *Marital separation.* New York: Basic Books.

Whelan, J. P., Meyers, A. W., & Elkin, T. D. (1996). Ethics in sport and exercise psychology. In J. L. Van Raalte & B. W. Brewer (Eds.), *Exploring sport and exercise psychology* (pp. 431–447). Washington, DC: American Psychological Association.

Wiese-Bjornstal, D. (1997). Psychological Dimensions. In *Physical activity & sport in the lives of girls: Physical and mental health*

dimensions from an interdisciplinary approach (pp. 17–35). Rockville, MD: SAMHSA.

Wiggins, J. G. (1996). Stress, behavioral physiology, capitation and the future of psychology. *The Independent Practitioner, 16,* 126–128.

Wildenhaus, K. J. (1997). Sport psychology services in a clinical practice. In L. VandeCreek, S. Knapp, & T. L. Jackson (Eds.), *Innovations in clinical practice: A source book, 15,* (pp. 365–383). Sarasota, FL: Professional Resource Press.

Wildman, T. J. (1998). Relational aspects of competition: A father learns from his daughters. In K. F. Hays (Ed.), *Integrating exercise, sports, movement, and mind: Therapeutic unity* (pp. 63–80). Binghamton, NY: Haworth.

Williams, J. M. (Ed.). 1998. *Applied sport psychology: Personal growth to peak performance* (3rd ed.). Mountain View, CA: Mayfield.

Williams, J. M., & Roepke, N. (1993). Psychology of injury and injury rehabilitation. In R. N. Singer, M. Murphey, & L. K. Tennant (Eds.), *Handbook of research on sport psychology* (pp. 815–839). New York: Macmillan.

Williams, J. M., & Straub, W. F. (1998). Sport psychology: Past, present, future. In J. M. Williams (Ed.), *Applied sport psychology: Personal growth to peak performance* (3rd ed., pp. 1–12). Mountain View, CA: Mayfield.

Wilson, G. T., & Eldredge, K. L. (1992). Pathology and development of eating disorders: Implications for athletes. In K. D. Brownell, J. Rodin, & J. H. Wilmore (Eds.), *Eating, body weight and performance in athletes: Disorders of modern society* (pp. 115–127). Philadelphia: Lea & Febiger.

Wilson, R. R. (1996). *Don't panic: Taking control of anxiety attacks.* New York: HarperPerennial.

Yambor, J. (1997, September). Lessons learned the hard way in sport psychology consulting. [Abstract]. *Journal of Applied Sport Psychology 8, [Suppl.]*, S174.

Yambor, J., & Connelly, D. (1991). Issues confronting female sport psychology consultants working with male student-athletes. *The Sport Psychologist, 5*, 304– 312.

Yates, A. (1991). *Compulsive exercise & the eating disorders: Toward an integrated theory of activity*. New York: Brunner-Mazel.

Zaichkowsky, L. D., & Perna, F. M. (1996). Certification in sport and exercise psychology. In J. L. Van Raalte & B. W. Brewer (Eds.), *Exploring sport and exercise psychology* (pp. 395–411). Washington, DC: American Psychological Association.

Zimmerman, T. S., Protinsky, H. O., & Zimmerman, C. S. (1994). Family systems consultation with an athletic team: A case study of themes. *Journal of Applied Sport Psychology, 6*, 101–115.

Author Index

Abrams, D. B., 40
Acevedo, E. O., 25
Agurs, T. D., 164
Airhihenbuwa, C. O., 164, 165
Alford, B. A., 25
Allison, D. B., 169
Allison, M. T., 158
Altshul, V. A., 67
American Psychiatric Association, 75, 76
American Psychological Association, 24,
    61, 175, 203, 205, 207, 208, 218, 240,
    241
Andersen, M. B., 25, 161, 163, 177, 178,
    187, 213
Antoni, M. H., 149
Arce, J. C., 159
Association for the Advancement of
    Applied Sport Psychology, 213
Auchus, M. P., 122, 130, 131, 135

Bacon, V. L., 158
Bahr, J. M., 65
Bahrke, M. S., 103
Bányai, É. I., 30
Barbach, L., 156, 159
Barlow, D. H., 92
Barnes, L., 59
Barrow, J. C., xiii
Beck, A., 49
Benshoff, J. J., 120
Benson, H., 103
Bergandi, T. A., 111

Berger, B. G., xiv, 7, 12, 13, 14, 16, 49, 50,
    55, 68, 69, 97, 98, 103, 104, 145, 168,
    196, 212, 213
Berne, E., 42
Beumont, C. C., 116
Beumont, P. J. V., 116
Biddle, S., 168
Birkimer, J. C., 7
Birnie, W. A., 130
Birrell, S., 17, 161, 165
Blais, M., 158
Bloom, M., 143
Blumenthal, J. A., 156, 173, 174
Bordo, S., 108, 115
Borg, G., 50
Bosscher, R. J., 81
Brackenridge, C. H., 186
Braden, C. J., 150
Brawley, L. R., 7, 8
Bredemeier, B. J. L., 30, 155
Brewer, B. W., 13, 177, 180, 209
Brewerton, T. D., 115
Brodsky, A. M., 68, 187
Brown, C. H., 29
Brown, D. R., 32, 208, 210
Brown, J. D., 98, 171
Brown, L. S., 137, 143, 187
Brown, P., 27, 63, 81
Brown, R. S., 13
Brown, S. A., 119, 120
Brown, T., 120
Brownell, K. D., 111, 112, 115, 181, 182

Brubaker, P. H., 98, 101, 164
Bruch, H., 114
Brustad, R. J., 29
Buffone, G. W., 13, 14, 37, 60, 61, 63
Bunker, L. K., 159, 170
Burke, K. L., 219
Burks, R., xiii
Butcher, L. A., 139
Butki, B. D., 161, 163
Byrne, A., 6
Byrne, D. G., 7

Cabaj, R. P., 163
Calfas, K. J., xiii
Campagna, P. D., 129, 130, 132, 134, 135
Carlton, E. B., 17
Carmack, M. A., 12
Carr, C. M., 29, 180
Casper, R. C., 114
Cerny, J. A., 92
Clayton, P. J., 87, 92
Claytor, R. P., 99, 169
Coakley, J., 180
Cochrane, C. E., 115
Cogan, K. D., 13, 24, 29, 154, 155, 158,
    161, 162, 163, 165, 177, 178, 179,
    185, 187, 206
Coleman, J. K., 23
Conn, V. S., 148
Connelly, D., 32, 187
Coppel, D. B., 29
Coster, J. S., xiii
Costill, D. L., 14
Courtois, C. A., 71, 143, 186
Cousins, S. O., 159
Cox, R. H., 26, 240
Cox, S., 7
Crandall, R. C., 6, 126, 159, 168
Crowther, J. H., 118
Csikszentmihalyi, M., 7, 151, 170

Damarajian, N., 187, 206, 217
Danish, S. J., 26, 122, 126, 214
Darling, N., 172
Davis, C., 115, 181
Davis, J. C., 54
DeAngelis, T., 156
DeBon, M., 164
DeMichele, J. T., 25
Denson, E. L., 177
De Souza, M. J., 159
DiClemente, C. C., 38, 44, 53, 245

Diehl, N. S., 206
Dishman, R. K., 45, 50, 53, 54, 55, 155
Donoghue, P. J., 150
Droppleman, L. F., 8
Duda, J., 155
Duivenvoorden, H. J., 148
Duncan, M. C., 158, 164
Dunlap, G., 169
Duquin, M. E., 30

Eaton, M., 103
Eccles, J. S., 158
Edmonson, K., 118
Edwards, S., 90, 103
Eischens, R. R., 79
Eldredge, K. L., 181, 182, 183
Elkin, T. D., 203
Ellickson, K. A., 32, 208, 210
Ellis, A., 25
English, T., xiii
Enns, C. Z., 143
Epling, W. F., 116
Epstein, L. H., 29, 170
Erickson, M. H., 57

Faigenbaum, A. D., 133
Fairburn, C. G., 113
Faith, M. S., 169
Fallon, P., 118
Faris, J., 79
Fawcett, J., 83
Feldman, R. H., xiii
Fender, L. K., 200
Fillingim, R. B., 173, 174
Fine, A. H., 170, 171
Fisher, E., 160
Fitzpatrick, M., 209, 211, 212, 213
Fletcher, M. A., 149
Flynn, M. G., 14
Foreyt, J. P., 110
Fosshage, J. L., 65
Foster, S., 31
Fox, J., 115
Franklin, R. D., 169
Freedson, P., 159, 170
Freud, A., 59
Freudenberger, H. J., 196
Freyd, J. J., 63, 137
Friedman, E., 103

Gallwey, W. T., 26
Garner, D. M., 113, 118

Gauvin, L., 102, 195
Gelinas, D., 71
Gill, D. L., 26, 30, 67, 153, 155, 160, 161
Gill, K., 156, 159
Glasser, W., 25, 120, 197
Gleser, J., 27, 63, 81
Godin, G., 54
Goldston, S. E., 4
Gologor, E., 63
Gomer, S., 219
Goode, E., 6
Goodman, A. S., 111
Goodrick, G. K., 110
Gordon, S., 176
Gorely, T., 176
Gorski, T. T., 45
Gould, D., 187, 206, 217, 219
Gratch, S. E., 17, 18, 155, 156
Green, B. S., 27, 104
Greenberg, D., 158
Greist, J. H., 13, 79, 121
Grembowski, D., 173
Griffin, J., 164, 183
Guerin, J. J., 139
Gurman, A. S., 79

Hale, B. D., 26, 214
Halgin, R. P., xiii, xv
Hall, R. L., 53, 165
Haney, C. J., 103
Harold, R. D., 158
Harris, B. L., 143
Harris, D. V., 143
Harris, M. B., 183
Hays, K. F., 14, 29, 30, 62, 63, 64, 65, 71,
    93, 139, 144, 206, 207, 210, 211, 212,
    220
Heil, J., 107, 110, 111, 151, 173, 180
Heitner, K., 175
Hellstedt, J. C., 29
Hendricks, G., 27
Henschen, K., 107, 110, 111, 173, 180,
    192, 200
Herman, J. L., 63, 68, 71, 137, 138, 141,
    142, 186
Heyman, S. R., 161, 162, 163
Heyward, V. H., 164
Hibbs, N., 115
Hill, K. L., 29, 30, 67, 154
Hodgdon, J. A., 6
Hodges, E. L., 115
Hoffart, A., 80, 122

Hoffman, P., 123, 194
Hollander-Goldfein, B., 65
Hollon, S., 49
Holmes, D. S., 83
Horn, T. S., 99, 169
Huang, C. A., 27
Hutchinson, D. S., 129, 133

Ironson, G., 149

Jabine, L. N., 114
Jaffee, L., 164
Janoff-Bulman, R., 138
Johnsgard, K. W., 8, 9, 14, 49, 52, 56, 60,
    61, 63, 68, 79, 100, 105, 121, 157
Jones, E., 6
Jordan, M. R., 57

Kabat-Zinn, J., 27, 94
Kahn, A. P., 83
Kaplan, H., 53
Kaslow, N., 122, 130, 131, 135
Kaslow, N. J., 130, 135
Kavussanu, M., 7, 90, 102
Keeley, S., xiii
Keita, G. P., 83
Kern, L., 169
Kirkcaldy, B. D., 7
Kirschenbaum, D. S., 50, 110, 111, 112
Klein, M. H., 7, 79
Klesges, R. C., 164
Klimas, N. G., 149
Koegel, R. L., 169
Koeppl, P. M., 109
Kostrubala, T., 14, 18, 60, 66, 211
Kremer, D., 120
Kroll, J., 66
Kruskemper, G. M., 148
Kugler, J., 148
Kumanyika, S., 164
Kunz, J. L., 180

LaMarche, J. A., 29
Lamont-Mills, A., 29, 154
Landers, D. M., 51, 90
LaPerriere, A., 149
Larkin, D., 168
Leffingwell, T., 218
Lendl, J., 31
Lenskyj, H., 155
Lerner, M., 148
Lesyk, J. J., 13, 50, 95, 220

Levine, M. D., 162
Levy, A. S., 109
Lewis, L. W., 111
Linder, D. E., 13, 177
Liu, Z., 26, 240
Long, B. C., 90, 101, 103
Long, B. J., xiii
Lorr, M., 8
Lowe, A., 164
Lox, C. L., 149
Lutter, J. M., 164
Lynch, J., 27, 143

McAuley, E., 7, 50, 102, 149
McCann, I. L., 141, 142, 145
McCann, L., 83
McCann, S., 192, 200
McClain, T. M., 98
McCullagh, P., 37, 78, 217
McDonald, D. G., 6
McEntee, D. J., xiii, xv
McGarvey, W. E., 109
McGlone, K., 150
McGowan, R. W., 84
McGrath, E., 83, 156
McInman, A., 7, 68
MacKenzie, M. M., 14
McKnight, J., 25, 26
McNair, D. M., 8
Mahoney, M. J., xiii, 178
Malkin, M. J., 120
Marcus, B. H., 38, 39, 40, 41, 43, 44, 45, 125, 148
Marlatt, G. A., 120
Martens, R., 12
Martin, S. B., 25, 26, 31
Martins, P., 53
Martinsen, E. W., 76, 78, 80, 81, 82, 83, 85, 122, 132, 134
Maslach, C., 196
Maslow, A. H., 9, 10
Mathews, A., 90, 103
May, J. R., 178, 240
Mehlenbeck, R. S., 23
Meichenbaum, D. H., 8, 55
Menapace, N., 30
Meyers, A. W., 23, 25, 164, 203
Miller, H. S., 98, 101, 164
Miller, W. R., 119, 120
Mitchell, J. E., 118
Mondin, G. W., 76, 195
Mooney, D. K., 154, 179, 193, 206

Morgan, D. L., 111
Morgan, L. K., 164
Morgan, W. P., 3, 4, 7, 8, 14, 30, 79, 81, 83, 103, 178, 196, 197, 200
Morris, M., 195
Moses, J., 90, 103
Murphey, M., 219
Murphy, M., 7, 27
Murphy, S., 25
Murphy, S. M., 13, 29, 62, 180, 181, 182
Murphy, T. J., 120
Murray, M., 163

National Advisory Mental Health Council, 129
Nellen, V. C., 122, 126
Nelson, M. B., 30, 161, 186, 212
Newman, J. R., 98
Niaura, R. S., 40
Noble, J. M., 217
Norcross, J. C., 25, 38, 44, 53, 245
Norris, J. L., 102
North, T. C., 31, 37, 78
Nulsen, J. C., 159

O'Connor, P. J., 14, 54, 178
Oglesby, C. A., 29, 30, 31, 67, 154, 158
O'Hanlon, W. H., 31
Orwin, A., 92
Ossip-Klein, D. J., 7
Overdorf, V., 159
Owen, D. R., 13, 49, 196
Owens, S. S., 122, 126

Pagano, R. R., 120
Pargman, D., 14
Pate, R. R., 178
Pearlman, L. A., 141, 142, 145
Pelham, T. W., 129, 130, 132, 134, 135
Pender, N. J., xiii
Pennington, F., 150
Perlman, S. G., 150
Perna, F. M., 207, 218
Petitpas, A., 26, 209, 213, 214
Petrie, T. A., 13, 24, 29, 154, 155, 158, 161, 162, 163, 165, 177, 179, 180, 182, 185, 206, 217
Petruzello, S. J., 51, 90
Pierce, E. F., 84
Pierce, R. A., 177
Pierce, W. D., 116
Pillow, D. R., 13, 177

Pincus, H. A., 75
Pinkerton, R. S., xiii
Pinto, B. M., 148, 165
Pool, J., 148
Pope, K. S., 137, 143, 186
Powell, R. R., 173
Powers, J. M., 120
Pretty, G. M. H., 29, 154
Prior, J. C., 156
Prochaska, J. O., 38, 39, 40, 41, 42, 43, 44, 45, 53, 245
Protinsky, H. O., 29
Puhl, J. L., 159

Qiu, Y., 26, 240

Raglin, J. S., 7, 14, 66, 87, 90, 91, 192, 194, 196, 197, 198
Rakowski, W., 38
Ramirez, D. E., 13
Ravizza, K., 187
Reed, C., 151
Rejeski, W. J., 6, 98, 100, 101, 102, 129, 164, 239
Reno, R. R., 13, 177
Report of the Ethics Committee, 212
Reynolds, F., 28
Rich, F., 75, 179
Rindskopf, K. D., 17, 18, 155, 156
Ritter-Taylor, M., 29
Ritvo, P. G., 130
Rivera, P., 209
Robison, J. I., 8
Rodgers, W. M., 7, 8
Rodin, J., 7, 107, 108, 109, 113, 115, 181, 182
Roepke, N., 197
Rogers, M. A., 8
Rose, B., 168
Rossi, E. L., 57
Rossi, J. S., 38, 40, 44
Rossi, S. I., 57
Rostant, L., 120
Rotella, R. J., 163
Royak-Schaler, R., xiii
Rudolph, D. L., 50
Rush, J., 49
Russo, N. F., 83
Rutter, P., 68, 212, 213
Ryan, J., 182

Sachs, M. L., 10, 13, 14, 15, 60, 61, 62, 120, 142, 170, 171, 195, 197, 200, 206, 208, 210, 212, 213, 214, 219
Sacks, M. H., 13, 14, 26, 60
Sagal, M., 220
Sallis, J. F., xiii, 53, 155
Salmon, P., 195
Sanstead, M., 7, 12, 14, 37, 50, 60
Sass, M. L., 109
Schaap, D., 162
Schmelzer, G. L., 31
Schneiderman, N., 149
Schwebel, M., xiii
Seelbach, H., 148
Seheult, C., 26
Selby, V. C., 40
Seligman, M. E. P., 7
Selye, H., 98, 196
Seraganian, P., 6, 120, 223
Serlin, I., 30
Shaw, B., 49
Sheehan, G., 8, 9, 110, 121, 126, 149
Shephard, R. J., 7, 173
Sherman, R. T., 109, 115, 181
Sherwood, N. E., 118
Shipman, W. M., 169
Siegel, J. M., 98, 171
Siegel, M. E., 150
Silberstein, L. R., 108, 109
Silva, J. M., 184, 196, 198
Sime, W. E., 3, 7, 12, 13, 14, 18, 37, 47, 48, 50, 54, 60, 69, 77, 93, 147, 148
Simons, C. W., 7
Singer, R. N., 219, 239
Sinyor, D., 120
Skrinar, G. S., 129, 133, 134, 136
Smith, D., 209, 211, 212, 213
Smith, R. C., 172
Smith, R. E., 167, 196
Smith, R. J., 206, 220
Smoll, F. L., 167
Solberg, Ø., 80, 122
Sonstroem, R. J., 99, 100
Sparling, P. B., 178
Specker, S., 118
Stainback, R. D., 29
Stanghelle, J. K., 82
Stavel, R. V., 90
Steege, J. F., 156
Stein, J. M., 91
Steinberg, H., 195
Stellefson, E. J., 115
Stephenson, M. G., 109

Steptoe, A., 7, 90, 103
Stern, E. M., 30
Stevenson, J. S., 173
Stoever, S., 182
Straub, W. F., 5, 240
Strean, H. S., 26
Strean, W. B., 26, 170
Strickland, B. R., 83
Striegel-Moore, R. H., 108, 109
Suinn, R. M., 25, 178
Summers, J., 14, 110
Swoap, R. A., 181, 182
Sykes, E. A., 195
Szabo, A., 195

Taub, J. M., 13
Taylor, J., 141, 217
Taylor, S. G., 148
Tennant, L. K., 219
Thayer, R. E., 98
Thompson, A., 6, 98, 100, 101, 129, 164, 239
Thompson, C. L., 25, 26, 31
Thompson, J. K., 160, 181
Thompson, R. A., 65, 109, 115, 181
Topp, R., 173
Touyz, S. W., 116
Tran, Z. V., 37, 78
Tucker, R. S., 149
Turk, D. C., 8, 55
Turner, J., 148, 149
Túry, F., 30

Udry, E. M., 25
Unger, K. V., 129, 130, 133
United States Department of Health and Human Services, 6, 156

Van Dixhoorn, J., 148
Van Raalte, J. L., 13, 177, 187, 209, 217
Verhage, F., 148
Vigna, Y. M., 156

Waddell, T., 162
Wakefield, C., 151
Walsh, B. T., 113, 118
Wankel, L. M., 51, 53, 55, 56
Weinberg, R. S., 219
Weiner-Davis, M., 31
Weiss, M. R., 167
Weiss, R. S., 138
Whelan, J. P., 23, 25, 203, 209
White, R. A., 7, 27
Wiese-Bjornstal, D., 158, 160, 182
Wiggins, J. G., 3
Wildenhaus, K. J., 31, 220, 222
Wildman, T. J., 30
Williams, H., 116
Williams, J. M., 5, 197, 219, 240
Williams-Rice, B. T., 25
Wilson, G. T., 181, 182, 183
Wilson, R. R., 27
Wiman, P., 148
Wolstat, H., 14, 110
Wonderlich, S. A., 118
Wood, K., 122, 130, 131, 135
Woody, G. E., 120

Yambor, J., 32, 187
Yates, A., 65, 115, 192
Yelmokas, A. M., 129

Zaichkowsky, L. D., 207, 218
Zimmerman, C. S., 29
Zimmerman, T. S., 29
Zseni, A., 30

Subject Index

Active-alert hypnosis, 30
Activity anorexia, 116
Addiction model, excessive exercise, 196–198
Adherence, 54–57
  definition, 55
  epidemiological studies, 8
  and exercise monitoring, 55
  goal setting link, 56, 159
  and obesity, 111–112
  rates of, 8, 55
Adolescents
  eating disorders, athletes, 181–184
  case example, 172–173
  female gender role stereotypes, 157–159
  practitioner recommendations, 173
  stress-coping methods, girls, 171–172
The Adventure Network, 121
Aerobic exercise
  alcohol abuse recovery, 120
  anxiety therapy, 90
  depressed inpatients, 80–81, 130
  elderly, 174
  HIV-positive patients, 149
  and meditation, 104
  premenstrual dysphoria benefits, 156
  psychiatric inpatients, 132, 134
  relaxation comparison, depression, 83
  in stress management, 103–104
Affirmations, 143
African Americans, 163–165
  body image, female adolescents, 164

hypertension risk, 164
role conflicts, females, 164–165
Agoraphobia, 91–92
Alcohol abuse, 119–124
  athletes, 180
  case example, 122–124
  comorbidity, 119
  practitioner recommendations, 126–127
  primary prevention, 122
  running therapy, 120–122
Amenorrhea, 159
American Psychological Association
Division of Exercise and Sport Psychology, 240–241
  ethical principles, 203–204, 213
Anorexia, 114–117
  athletes, 180–184
  case example, 114–115
  comorbid conditions, 118
  excessive exercise, 115–116
  practitioner recommendations, 116–117
Antidepressants, 75–76
  and exercise, 81–82
  inpatients' evaluation of, 81
  side effects, 75–76
  and women, 83
Anxiety, 87–95
  case examples, 87–89, 93
  conceptual issues, 90
  depression comorbidity, 87
  exercise deprivation effect, 195–196
  and exercise intensity, 90–91

practitioner recommendations, 94–95
prevalence, 87
walk-talk therapy, 93–94
Arousal management, trauma survivors,
140–141
Arthritis patients, 150
Asceticism, 115
Association for the Advancement of
Applied Sport Psychology
ethical principles, 203–204, 213
history, 240
Associative thinking
anxious thoughts redirection, 94
case example, 142–143
trauma survivors, 142–143
Athletes, 177–187
attitude toward psychotherapy, 13
confidentiality, 208–209
depression, 178–179
eating disorders, 180–184
emotional problems, 177–187
rates of, 178
family systems perspective, 29
phobic behavior, 184–185
and practitioner competence, 206
practitioner recommendations, 187
and sexual abuse, 185–187
sexual orientation conflicts, 161–163
substance abuse, 180
Attentional focus, 141–142
Autistic children, 169

Barriers to exercise, 54
Behavioral methods
effectiveness, 25
sport psychology relevance, 25
Behavioral physiology, 3
Behavioral processes, and change, 40,
43–44
Beliefs, assessment of, 51–52
Biomedical model, 6
Biopsychosocial model, 6
Bipolar disorder, 81
Blacks. *See* African Americans
Body cues, 63
Body image
ethnic differences, 164
and exercise during therapy, 67–68
gender role differences, 155
self-esteem interaction, 100
and strength training, women, 160
Body memories, 63

Body-mind relationship, 6
Bone mass, 159
Boredom, relapse predictor, 57
Boundaries, 209–213
crossing of, 209
and dual role relationships, 210–211
and exercise during therapy, 64–66, 210
physical contact, 212
and self-disclosure, 211–212
sexual contact, 212–213
violations of, 209
Breast cancer, 148–149
Breathing techniques
arousal management, 140–141
case study, 22
Bulimia, 112–114
athletes, 182
comorbid conditions, 118
excessive exercise, 113
practitioner recommendations, 113–114
vicious cycle in, 112–113
Burnout, 196–198
characteristics, 196
and excessive exercise, 196–197

Caloric expenditure, and obesity, 110
Cancer, 148–149
Cardiac rehabilitation, 148
Cardiovascular fitness
hospitalized schizophrenics, 129–130
mentally ill undergraduates, 133
Cardiovascular prescription, 50
"Certified Consultant, AAASP," 207, 218
Change process, 37–45
FIT concept as measure, 51
stages of, 37–45
transtheoretical model, 37
Children, 168–171
developmental factors, 168
obesity, 169–170
parental involvement, 170–171
physical coordination effects, 168–169
practitioner recommendations, 171
self-esteem, 169
Chronic fatigue syndrome, 150–151
Chronic mental illness, 129–136
exercise benefits, 129–133
medication concern, 133–134
patient's perspective, 134–135
practitioner recommendations, 135–136
rate of, 129
Chronic pain, 160

Clients, 11–19
Coaches
    attitudes toward weight, 183–184
    and dual role relationships, 210
    parental interaction, children, 170–171
    sexual exploitation by, 185–187
    therapist's confidentiality, 209
Cognitive-behavioral methods
    effectiveness, 25
    sport psychology relevance, 25
Cognitive functioning, elderly, 173
Community psychology, 29
Competence, 204–207
Competition, 67
Compliance, 54–55. *See also* Adherence
Compulsive exercise. *See* Overuse
Confidentiality, 207–209
    and coaches, 209
    and exercise during therapy, 66
    and high-performance athletes, 208
    as "primary obligation," 207
Consultant role, 15–16, 217–218
Coping ability
    adolescent girls, 171–172
    aerobic training benefits, 91, 103–104
    exercise immediate and long-term
        effects, 100–102
Coronary patients, 148
Cross-training, 200
Cultural context, 153–165, 206

Dance therapy, 30
Decisional Balance Scale, 41, 245
Depression, 75–85
    adolescent girls, 158
    athletes, 178–179
    case examples, 43–45, 76–77
    change stages, case examples, 43–45
    costs, 75
    elderly, 174
    goal setting, 85
    inpatient setting, 80–81, 130, 132
    and medical illness, 148–149
    medication treatment, 75–76, 81–82
    meta-analysis, exercise studies, 78–79
    practitioner recommendations, 84–85
    psychotherapy versus exercise, 79–81
    rates of, 75
    in women, 82–84
Developmental counseling model, 26
Diaphragmatic breathing, 94
Diary record, 55

Diet concerns, and gender, 108–109
Dissociative thinking
    anxious thoughts redirection, 94
    case example, 142–143
    trauma survivors strategy, 142–143
Distress, 98
Diversity issues, 153–165
Dose of exercise, 50–51
    and mood, 194–196
    prescription, 50–51
Dragons Abreast, 148–149
Dropouts, 55. *See also* Adherence
Drug abuse, 119–124
    athletes, 180
    case example, 122–124
    comorbidity, 119
    practitioner recommendations,
        126–127
    primary prevention, 122
    running therapy, 121
Drug "holidays," 134
Dual role relationships
    case example, 210–211
    complexity of, 210–211
    exercise during therapy danger, 64–65,
        210
Dualism legacy, 5–6
Duke Aging and Exercise Study, 173
Duration of exercise, 50–51

Eastern philosophy, 26–28
Eating disorders, 107–118
    anorexia, 114–117
    athletes, 159, 180–184
    bulimia, 112–114
    exercise during therapy risk, 65
    gender issues, 108–109
    mixed diagnosis, 117–118
Education, 215–223
Elderly, 173–176
    case example, 175
    cognitive function, 173
    hypochondriasis, 175
    practitioner recommendations, 176
    women, 159
Endogenous opioids, 123, 194
Endorphins, 123, 194
Environmental factors, 54
Ethical issues, 203–214
    boundaries, 209–213
    and competence, 204–207
    confidentiality, 207–209

and diagnosis, 213–214
exercise during psychotherapy, 61
Ethnicity, 163–165
female role conflicts, 164–165
practitioner recommendations, 165
and therapist's competence, 206
Eustress, 98
Exercise addiction. *See* Overuse
The Exercise and Sport Psychology
Development Plan, 31–33, 215,
229–235
Exercise deprivation, 195–196
Exercise during psychotherapy, 59–71
benefits, 13–14, 60–61
body awareness aspect, 63–64
boundary maintenance, 64–65,
210–212
characteristics and issues, 60–64
client issues, 65
and dual role relationships, 210
ethical principles, 61–62, 210–212
interpersonal issues, 64–68
risks, 61
running approach, 70–71
and self-disclosure, 211–212
sexual abuse survivors, 69–71
and sexuality, 67–68
supervision, 61
therapist issues, 62–63, 66
walk-talk approach, 68–70
Exercise history
importance in exercise planning,
51–52
interview assessment, 244
Exercise History, Motivation Inventory,
and Exercise Plan, 48, 243–246
Experiential perspective, 26–28, 40
Eye Movement Desensitization and
Reprocessing, 313

Family systems, 28–29
and athletes, 29
case example, 28–29
team functioning link, 29
Fees, 221–222
Feldenkrais, 30
"Female athlete triad," 159
Femininity, meaning of, 155
Feminism, 29–30
FIT acronym, 50–51
as change measure, 51
and trauma survivors, 144–145

Flashbacks, 63
Frequency of exercise, 50
Functional Integration, 30

Gay Games, 162
Gay men, 161–163
gender identity issues, 162–163
practitioner recommendations, 163
Gender differences
depression, 82–83
and exercise during therapy, 67
exercise socialization, 52–53
weight and diet concerns, 108–109
Gender roles
adolescent girls, 157–159
conflicts, 158
African American women, 165
and exercise socialization, 17–18,
154–155, 160
Gestalt therapy, 28–29
Goal Attainment Scaling, 31
Goal setting
adherence link, 56, 159
depression, 85
and exercise maintenance, 56
trauma survivors, 144
Graduate education, 218–219
Grief, and walk-talk therapy, 77
Griffith, Coleman, 239
Group activity, 53
Group psychotherapy, 18
Guided imagery, 143
Gymnasts, 29, 182, 185

Hatha yoga, 94
Health clearance, depressed patients, 84
Hindu power, 27
HIV-positive patients, 149
Holism, 21
Homonegativity, 161–163
Hypertension risk, Blacks, 164
Hypnosis, 30
Hypochondriasis, 175

Incest survivors. *See* Sexual abuse
survivors
Inpatient setting, depression, 80–81
Intensity of exercise
anxiety therapy, 90–91
and mood, 194–196
obese children, 170
prescription for, 50–51

Interoceptive exposure, 92–95

Jogging
  children, 169
  psychotherapeutic benefits, 13–14
  in psychotherapy, 60
Journal of Applied Sport Psychology, 219
Journal of Exercise and Sport Psychology, 219
Judo principles, 27–28

Lesbians, 161–163
  gender identity issues, 162–163
  practitioner issues, 163
  sexual abuse, female coaches, 186
Liability issues, 66, 207
Life span, 167–176
  adolescents, 171–173
  children, 168–171
  developmental model, 26
  elderly, 159, 173–176
Life stress
  adolescent girls, coping, 171–172
  depression prevention, women, 84
Life-style revision, 44–45
Log record, 55, 112
Long-term goals, 56
Low-back pain, 150

Maintenance of exercise
  as change stage, 44
  goal setting importance in, 56
  pragmatics, 47–58
Marketing, 215–223
Martial arts, 27–28
Masculinity, meaning of, 155
Mastery
  definition, 100
  exercise long-term effects, 101–102
  exercise program recommendations, 105
Medical illness, 147–152
Medical model, 6
Medications
  chronic mental illness, 133–134
  depression treatment, 75–76, 81–82
Meditation
  action incorporation, 27
  exercise combination, 103–104
  versus psychotherapy, depression, 79–80
  in stress management, 103–104
Men, exercise socialization, 52
Menopausal women, 156
Mental illness, chronic, 129–136

Mental rehearsal, 143
Metaphoric representation, 63
Mind-body connection, 5–7
Monitoring exercise, 55
Mood
  exercise benefits, 8
  exercise criteria, taxonomy, 49
  and exercise dose, 194–196
  ratings of, 84
Motivation
  changes over time, 56–57
  interview assessment, 243–246

Narrative therapy, 31
Neuro-Linguistic Programming, 30
Non-verbal communication, 63

Obesity
  case example, 109–110
  in children, 169–170
  and exercise adherence, 111–112
  exercise role, 110–112
  practitioner recommendations, 111–112
  women's stigmatization, 109
Obsessive-compulsive clients, 65, 95
Obsessive exercise. See Overuse
Optimism, and regular exercise, 102
Osteoporosis, 156, 159
Overuse, 191–201
  addiction model, 196–197
  and anorexia, 114–116
  and bulimia, 113
  and burnout, 196–197
  case examples, 193–194, 198–199
  exercise deprivation effects, 195
  physiological basis, 116, 196
  practitioner recommendations, 200–201
  psychosocial costs, 191–193
  remediation, 198–200
  stress model, 196
Overweight. See Obesity

Pain patients, 150–151
Panic disorder
  case examples, 87–89, 91
  depression comorbidity, 87
  exercise therapy, 91–92
  vigorous exercise precipitation of, 91
Parental involvement, 170–171
Perceived effort, 50
Phenothiazine medication, 134
Phobic behavior, athletes, 184–185

Physical activity
  definition, 4
  client's history of, 32–33
Physical fitness, and mental illness,
  129–130
Physical illness, 147–152
Play, 9
Play therapy, 59
"Positive addiction," 121, 197
Postdoctoral training, 219
Posttraumatic stress disorder. *See* Trauma
  survivors
Power issues, 67
Practice competence, 205–206
Premenstrual syndrome, 156
Pro bono work, 222
Professional athletes. *See* Athletes
Profile of Mood States, 8, 84, 178
Program adherence. *See* Adherence
Psychiatric inpatients, 80–81
Psychoanalytic theory, 25–26
Psychoeducational approach, 25
Psychosomatic, 3
Psychotherapists. *See* Therapists
Psychotherapy during exercise. *See* Exercise
  during psychotherapy
Psychotherapy versus exercise, depression,
  79–80
Psychotic depression, 81
Psychotropic medication. *See* Medications
Pygmalion effect, 18

Questionnaire on Exercise, xiii

Ratings of Perceived Exertion scale, 50
Rational-emotive methods, 25
Reality therapy, 25
Recreational exercisers, 12
Referral sources, 220–221
Relapse, 57–58
  case example, 57–58
  and change stages, 45
  predictors, 57
Relaxation training
  case study, 22
  versus exercise, depression, 83
  versus psychotherapy, depression, 79–80
  trauma survivors, 140–141
Remediation, excessive exercise, 198–200
Resistance, 26
Resting metabolic rate, 110
Rheumatoid arthritis, 150

Right-brain thinking, 62
Role model, therapist as, 17–18
"The runner's high," 10, 194
Running
  addiction model, 197
  alcohol and drug abuse recovery,
    120–121
  depressed inpatients, 81
  during therapy, 61, 64, 70–71, 211
    case examples, 70–71, 211–212
  and interoceptive exposure, 92, 95
  and meditation, 27
  motivational changes over time, 56
  in panic disorder, 92, 95
  smoking incompatibility, 126
  therapist's participation, 18–19
  as therapy, 13–14
  verbal therapy comparison, 13
Running addiction, 197–200
Running deprivation, and mood, 195

Schizophrenia, 129–136
  exercise benefits, 132
  medication concerns, 133–134
  patient's perspective, 134–135
  physical fitness deficits, 129–130
  practitioner recommendations, 135–136
Selective serotonin reuptake inhibitors, 76,
  82
Self-actualization, 9–10
Self-concept
  definition, 99
  exercise benefits, 7
Self-disclosure, 66
Self-efficacy
  adolescent girls, 172
  and change process, 41
Self-esteem, 97–105
  and body image, 100
  children, 169–170
  definition, 99
  exercise immediate and long-term
    effects, 100–102
  exercise interactions, 99–100
  practitioner recommendations, 105
Set point, 110
Sex differences. *See* Gender differences
Sexual abuse survivors
  adventure challenge programs, 139
  associative and dissociative strategies,
    142–143
  athletes, 185–187

attentional focus, 141–142
case examples, 70–71, 139–143
running therapy, case example, 70–71
walk-talk therapy, 69–70
Sexual contact, 212–213
Sexual orientation, 161–163
Sexuality, and exercise during therapy, 67
Short-term goals, 56
Siddhi, 27
SMART acronym, 56
Smoking cessation, 124–126
case example, 124–125
running therapy, 126
Social supports, 53
Socialization, gender differences, 52–53
Sociocultural variables, 52–53, 153–165
Solution-focused therapy, 31
Somatopsychic, 3, 147
The Sport Psychologist, 219
Sport psychology
cognitive-behavioral and behavioral
methods, 25
definition, 5
education and training, 216–219
Eastern and experiential perspectives,
26–28
feminist perspective, 29–30
history, 239–241
organizations, 240
psychodynamic theory relevance, 25–26
theoretical perspectives, 24–31
and therapist competence, 205–207
Sports teams, systems perspective, 29
Stage theory, 38–40
Staleness model, 196–197
Stereotypes, 152–165
ethnicity, 163–165
and sexual orientation, 161–163
women, 153–161
Strength training, women, 160
Stress
adolescent girls, 171–172
aerobic training benefits, 90–91,
102–104
definitional issues, 98–100
depression prevention, women, 84
exercise as buffer, 98
Stress management, 102–105
Substance abuse, 119–127
alcohol and drug abuse, 119–124
athletes, 180
practitioner recommendations, 126–127

primary prevention, 122
smoking, 124–126
Supervision, 61
Supportive role, psychotherapist, 16
Symbolic representations, 63
Systemic lupus erythematosus, 150
Systems perspective, 28–29
and athletes, 29
case example, 28–29

Talk test, 50
Tao philosophy, 27
Team functioning, 29
Therapeutic Recreators for Recovery,
121
Therapists, 11–19
competence, 204–207
consultant role, 15–16
ethics, 203–214
exercise during therapy benefits to,
62–63
exercise patterns, xiii–xvi
hubris factor, 207
as participants, 18–19
sport-related practice, survey, 23
Third-party payment, 213–214
Thought Field Therapy, 30
Touch, 212
Training, 215–223
Trait anxiety, 90, 102
Transference, 26
Transtheoretical model, 38
Trauma survivors
adolescent girls, 158
adventure challenge programs, 139
arousal management, 140–141
associative and dissociative strategies,
142–143
attentional focus, 141
case examples, 69–70, 139–142
empowerment, 137–146
exercise therapy approach, 63,
138–140
FIT concept application, 144–145
goal setting, 144
practitioner recommendations, 145–146
transitional objects, 143–144
visualization techniques, 143
walk-talk therapy, 69–70
Triathletes
case example, 198–200
exercise addiction, 198–200

Tricyclic antidepressants, 134

Visual Motor Behavioral Rehearsal, 25
Visualization, trauma survivors, 143

Walk-talk therapy, 60, 68–70
    advantages, 60, 68–69
    in anxiety, 93–94
    case examples, 69–70, 76–77
    in depression, 76–77
    psychological value, 60
    traditional psychotherapy difference,
        18–19
Walking
    anorexic clients, 116
    chronic mental patients, 135
    and group psychotherapy, 18
    and meditation, 27
    obese children, 170
Weight control
    athletes, 180–184
    coaches' attitudes, 183–184
Weight lifting, 131, 135
Weight loss, 109–111
    case example, 109–110
    maintenance of, 110–111

practitioner recommendations, 111–112
program adherence, 111–112
women's preoccupation, 108–110
Weight training, women, 160
Well-being, 3–10
Withdrawal from exercise, 197
Women, 153–161
    adults and elderly, 159
    and depression, 82–84
    eating disorders, 108–109
        athletes, 159, 180–184
    exercise socialization, 52–53, 154–155
    minority group role conflicts, 165
    physical benefits of exercise, 155–156
    practitioner recommendations, 160–161
    psychological benefits of exercise,
        156–157
    and sociability, 157
    underappreciation of exercise, 155
    weight concerns, 108–110
Women's Sports Foundation, 155
Wrestlers, weight control, 182–183

Yoga
    in anxiety, 94
    elderly clients, 174–175

About the Author

Kate F. Hays, PhD, practiced psychology in the United States for 25 years, incorporating sport psychology into her clinical practice. Now in Toronto, she continues to explore the relationship between mind and body in her consulting practice, The Performing Edge. Dr. Hays supports clients' use of exercise and provides performance enhancement training to athletes, performing artists, and business people. She brings additional personal energy and creativity to this work through her own involvement as a runner and musician.

Dr. Hays also focuses on training mental health professionals in sport, exercise, and performance. Her writings and lectures target these fields. She edited *Integrating Exercise, Sports, Movement, and Mind: Therapeutic Unit* (Haworth, 1998) and has written numberous articles and book chapters on the subject.

Dr. Hays is active as both a Fellow of the American Psychological Association (APA) and a Certified Consultant for the Association for the Advancement of Applied Sport Psychology. Dr. Hays served as Council Representative for the APA, chaired the APA's Board for the Advancement of Psychology in the Public Interest, and is currently president-elect of the APA's Division of Exercise and Sport Psychology.